PRACTICAL BURNS MANAGEMENT

PRACTICAL BURNS MANAGEMENT

J. V. Harvey Kemble
MA (Cantab), FRCS (Eng)

Consultant Plastic Surgeon, St. Bartholomew's Hospital, London,
and North East Thames Regional Plastic Surgery and Burns Centre,
St. Andrew's Hospital, Billericay, Essex

and

Brenda E. Lamb
SRN, ONC, DN (Lond)

Director of Nursing Services, (Acute Unit),
Basildon and Orsett Hospitals, Essex

HODDER AND STOUGHTON
LONDON SYDNEY AUCKLAND TORONTO

British Library Cataloguing in Publication Data

Kemble, J. V. Harvey
    Practical burns management.
    1. Burns and scalds——Treatment
    I. Title   II. Lamb, Brenda E.
    617'.1106   RD96.4

ISBN 0 340 36997 3

First published 1987

Typeset in Bembo by Tradespools Ltd, Frome, Somerset.

Printed and bound in Great Britain for Hodder and Stoughton Educational,
a division of Hodder and Stoughton Ltd, Mill Road, Dunton Green,
Sevenoaks, Kent by Richard Clay Ltd, Bungay, Suffolk

Additional Contributors

Rosamond M. Ford, DipCOT, SROT
  Lecturer in Occupational Therapy, Faculty of Sciences,
  Humanities and Community Studies, Colchester Institute,
  Colchester, Essex

Anthony C. Kaeser, MRCP (Lond), FRCPsych., DPM
  Consultant Psychiatrist, Basildon and Runwell Hospitals, Essex

Diana M. R. Swallow, MB, BS, FFARCS (Eng).
  Consultant Anaesthetist, Basildon and Thurrock District, Essex

'Fire and people do in this agree,
They both good servants, both ill masters be'.

Baron Brooke, Earl of Warwick. 1554–1628.

Contents

		Page
PREFACE		xiii
1	FIREMAKER MAN	1
2	AETIOLOGY, INCIDENCE, MORTALITY AND PREVENTION	
	Aetiology and incidence	4
	Mortality	8
	Prevention	8
3	SKIN AND PATHOPHYSIOLOGY OF THE BURN	
	Skin	11
	Circulation changes and fluid loss	13
	Gastro-intestinal tract	16
	The lungs	16
4	FIRST AID	
	Hot fluids and scalds	18
	Flame	18
	Chemical burns	19
	Electrical burns	21
	Inhalation injury	21
	Frostbite	22
	Transportation	22
5	ACCIDENT AND EMERGENCY DEPARTMENT MANAGEMENT	
	Preparation for arrival	24
	Safeguarding the airway	24
	Bleeding	25
	Analgesia	25
	Shock	25
	History	26
	Examination and records	26
	Assessment of the burn	28
	Wound cleaning	33

Inpatient management   33
Laboratory investigation   34
Intravenous fluid replacement   34
Escharotomy   36
Eyelids   38
Transfer from the accident department   38
Admission procedure   39

6 OUTPATIENT AND SURGERY MANAGEMENT
Diagnosis of burn depth   41
General treatment   41
Wound management   41

7 EARLY CARE IN THE DISTRICT GENERAL HOSPITAL
Reassessment of the burn injury   43
Wound cleaning   44
Dressing or wound exposure   44
Intravenous fluids   45
Continuing reassessment   48

8 FLUID AND ELECTROLYTE MANAGEMENT
Fluid loss   52
Water and electrolyte depletion   54
Acid–base equilibrium   57
Alternative IV replacement fluids   58

9 SHOCK: NURSING, MONITORING AND CHARTING
General impression   63
Respiration   64
Colour of skin and mucous membranes   65
Temperature   65
Pulse   65
Urine output   66
Central venous pressure   66

10 INFECTION AND WOUND MANAGEMENT
Wound care   68
Bath therapy   74
Dressing room   74
Analgesia   75
Partial thickness burns   75
Deep and full thickness burns   76
Skin grafts   76
Septicaemia   78
Hyperthermia   81

11 ELECTRICAL BURNS
Pathogenesis of electrical injury   83
Low tension injuries   85

High tension injuries   86
Electric arc burns   87
Lightning injuries   88

12 CHEMICAL BURNS
Acids   91
Alkalis   93
Sodium hypochlorite   94
Eyes   94
Metallic sodium, potassium and lithium   95
Phosphorus   95
Organic chemicals   95
Bitumen   96
Potassium permanganate   96
Cooking fat burns   96
Oesophageal burns   96
Bronchial burns   98

13 RADIATION BURNS
Pathogenesis   100
Radiation overdosage   100
Nuclear explosion   102

14 THE BURNS OPERATING THEATRE
The timing of grafting procedures   105
Preparation of splints   107
Immediate pre-operative preparation   107
The operation   108
Graft storage   110
Types of graft   110

15 ANAESTHESIA FOR THE BURNED PATIENT (*D.M.R. Swallow*)
General anaesthesia for excision and grafting procedures   115
General anaesthesia for excision of burns in children   119
Anaesthesia for dressings and minor procedures   122
Special conditions requiring early operation   122
Pain relief   123
General anaesthesia for late complications   124

16 INTENSIVE CARE OF THE PATIENT WITH RESPIRATORY BURNS
(*D.M.R. Swallow*)
Mechanisms of hypoxaemia associated with inhalational
damage   125
Recognition and diagnosis of the extent of the injury   127
Management   129
Additional respiratory complications in patients with burn
injury   136
Information from additional investigations   139

17   ACUTE RENAL FAILURE
     Prevention of renal failure   144
     Haemoglobinuria and myoglobinuria   144
     Established renal failure   145
     Haemodialysis   146
     Peritoneal dialysis   148

18   SPECIAL CONSIDERATIONS IN NURSING PAEDIATRIC BURN PATIENTS
     Different physical responses and needs   151
     Decreased co-operation   151
     Increased psychological trauma   152
     Different emotional needs   153
     Different cosmetic needs   154
     The needs of the parents and family   155
     Non-accidental injury   155
     Paediatric dosage   156

19   NUTRITION IN BURNS
     Protein loss   158
     Catabolic phase   158
     Calorific requirements   159
     Dietary control   159
     Sutherland and Batchelor charts   159
     Weights of common foods   160
     Composition of common foods   160
     Calculation of nitrogen losses   162
     Composition of milk   163
     Composition of enteral feeds   164
     Composition of supplementary feeds   164
     Average body weights   165

20   SCARS AND CONTRACTURES
     Prevention and minimizing scars and scar contracture   167
     Hypertrophic scarring   170
     Keloids   172
     Treatment of established contractures   173
     Long-standing scars   173

21   BURNS OF SPECIAL SITES
     Hands   175
     Ears   176
     Eyelids   176
     Mouth   176
     Face   177
     Neck   177

22   LATE SURGERY FOR BURNS
     Eyelids   180
     Eyebrows   181

Mouth 182
Nose 182
The neck 183
Axilla, antecubital fossa, popliteal fossa 183
Dorsum of foot and toes 184
The hand 184

23 PRACTICAL ASPECTS OF SPLINTAGE (*R.M. Ford*)
Indications for splintage 188
Materials and equipment 189
Splinting with exercise 190
Aftercare 190
Specific areas which may require splinting 191
Suppliers 209

24 THE BURNS TEAM AND UNIT
The multidisciplinary team 211
The nursing team in the burns unit 212
The burns unit 214
Location of the burns unit 216

25 PSYCHIATRIC ASPECTS OF BURN INJURY(*A.C. Kaeser*)
Obtaining psychiatric and psychological advice 219
Psychiatric aspects of the patient which contribute to the
burn injury 221
Psychological and psychiatric aspects during hospital stay 222
Psychological support in hospital and after discharge 226
Psychiatric aspects of the family in burned patients 227
Psychiatric and psychological aspects for nursing and
paramedical staff 229
Management of the violent burned patient 230
The burned child 231
The mentally handicapped 233
Social work 233
Post-traumatic neuroses and compensation claims 234
Relationships with the police 235

APPENDICES
Normal average values 238
Expected normal values of urine 239
Expected normal values of blood constituents 240
Conversion tables 242
Equipment 245
Hospitals with burn facilities 252
Poison centres for advice 255

INDEX 257

Preface

There are several excellent books about the burn injury on the market. Unfortunately for the hard-pressed casualty officer or nurse, duty registrar, intensive care staff or occasional burn surgeon in a District General Hospital, the practical management in many of them is often mingled with the research and academic considerations, making it difficult to extract vital information in a hurry.

With this in mind we offer a text where what is required from the attending surgeon, anaesthetist or nurse who has to treat these injuries intermittently, takes precedence over the more involved aspects of the contentious, theoretical or conjectural.

In such a work there is of course a danger of appearing dogmatic by implying that only one line of treatment is acceptable. Any such implication belies the facts encountered by specialists dealing daily with the burn injury. As quipped Oscar Wilde: 'Don't say you agree with me. When people agree with me I always feel I must be wrong'. The methods in this book, however, have all been tried and found to work well in practice. The doctor or nurse who uses them will be providing sound care for his patient, while acknowledging that there may be several other ways of achieving the same end.

From where do staff working in District General Hospitals gain knowledge to deal competently with severe burn injury? The subject is, on the whole, not taught in detail in most medical and nursing schools, and few will have ever treated these victims during preregistration training or the early years as a staff nurse.

Only a minority would have the ability and confidence to manage such an injury well. One's own 'experience teaches slowly, and at the cost of mistakes' (J.A. Froude, 1818–94). It is therefore essential to have at one's fingertips a book providing rapid and competent guidance to supplement advice given on the telephone or while more expert aid is arriving. This book aims to be that guide.

The book has been arranged in such a way that a course of treatment necessary at any one time after the burn accident can easily be found by reference to the relevant chapter, without having to read through the entire book up to that point.

As the practitioner becomes more expert we would hope he would wish to enlarge his knowledge of the subject as a whole, while we recognize that for some, half a dozen cases of severe burns per year may be the maximum he is likely to experience. With one or two exceptions, inserted to put the subject into context, we have therefore avoided the temptation to include details which although interesting and informative, are not directly related to the immediate practicalities of caring for a burn victim. With Winston Churchill, we have sought to avoid 'The tossing sea of Cause and Theory' in favour of 'the firm ground of Result and Fact'.

We acknowledge debts of gratitude to our colleagues for their interest, advice and criticism. Jean Green and Joanna Pons have typed the manuscript into intelligibility. Jack Bridger Chalker and Margot Cabel have created the line drawings with care and expertise. Janet Shugrue, District Dietician, has provided much of the data on nutrition.

We are grateful to Mrs Susan Devlin of our publishers Hodder and Stoughton for her sound, professional advice and assistance.

It is our hope that this introduction to the subject of the burn injury will be a source of assistance to hard-pressed doctors, nurses and therapists who find themselves called upon to treat a burned patient whose injuries are potentially devastating in their effect.

J.V.H.K.
B.E.L.

1

Firemaker Man

Fire has savaged man's ancestors since he appeared on Earth. Since before recorded history he has used fire for his own purposes. No doubt its benefits were first discovered by accident, but knowledge of its worth slowly spread.

Learning to control fire freed man from many of the restrictions imposed by his natural, and often hostile environment. About 400 000 years ago, *Homo erectus*, preceding *Homo sapiens*, found that he could choose to remain in regions previously denied to him by darkness (the depths of caves) or cold. He used fire to drive away dangerous carnivores, and to soften flesh to eat. Of the many primitive tribes who used fire, some knew how to make it, while others carefully nurtured fire-brands taken from neighbouring tribes.

The purposeful use of fire is very ancient. A yew-wood spear sharpened by Paleolithic man, its dip deliberately hardened by fire, has been discovered by archeologists in Saxony, in beds 100 000 years old; with it lay the skeleton of an extinct species of elephant whose death that spear may have caused.

Man has knowingly risked his life to reap the benefits which fire brings. Soon after 4000 BC men in Egypt found that by heating copper in furnaces, they could cast it into any desired shape. It could be given a cutting edge or fashioned into jewellery. From this momentous discovery, the whole of our modern technology has developed.

It is certain that Man has benefited from fire since the earliest times, but many have paid the price in suffering, scarring and even death. Doubtless the first healing applications for burns were leaves and grasses. By 5000 BC extracts from the barks and leaves of trees and shrubs were being used in China. Two thousand years later animal fats were being advocated in Egypt. Every century has seen the introduction of new applications, only some of which have stood the test of time. Vinegar, introduced by Galen, is still useful in the control of basophilic organisms such as *Pseudomonas aeruginosa*. Bull's gall and ashes of a dog's head are two of the many applications discarded over the ages.

Firstaiders and surgeons still advocate immediate cooling of the burned part with water. This treatment was recognized as being

1

useful as long ago as the ninth century by the Arabic physician, Rhases.

One of the early 'text books' devoted solely to burns which has come down to us is William Clowes' (1544–1604) *A Profitable and Necessarie Booke of Observations for All That are Burned with the Flames of Gunpowder* dated 1596 (now in the British Museum Library).

In Paris, Guillaume Dupuytren (1777–1835) described the different depths of burns (dividing them into six levels) and in 1842 Thomas Curling (1811–88) of the London Hospital drew attention to the gastric and duodenal ulceration which accompanies complicated burns injury.

The middle of the nineteenth century saw the concentration of expertise in one place in the opening of a Burns Unit in 1848 by James Syme (1799–1870) of Edinburgh. Forty years were to pass before the beneficial effect of treating the plasma circulatory losses by salt infusion was realized. This single advance has contributed more than any other to reducing the mortality from burns. Credit is due to von Lesser (1880) in Paris and H. von Tappeiner (1881) in Germany. Haldor Sneve (1905) of Minnesota and Alfred Blalock (1931) of Tennessee publicized this good practice.

It was not until 1942 that the full extent of the fluid loss from the circulation was appreciated, not only from the burned skin surface, but also into all the body interstitial space. Everett Evans of Richmond, Virginia, (1907–54) developed a formula for fluid replacement based on the patient's weight and the surface area burned; after adaptation, this became the Brooke Army formula.

Many serious burn injuries were prevented in naval ships during the First World War by the compulsory wearing of anti-flash hoods, gloves and overalls. The value of this was again demonstrated in the Falklands conflict of 1982.

Despite our 20th century disdain for the apparently unscientific remedies research has shown that many herbal remedies contain therapeutic properties. Tannic acid derived from tree bark was most effective in encouraging eschar formation in a burned wound. Its use was encouraged during the Second World War, and continued until 1944 when it was found to be connected with systemic absorption and hepatotoxicity.

Surgical principles were adapted and put to good effect by Archibald McIndoe (1900–1960) at East Grinstead, Sussex and Harry Brown of Indianapolis in the 1940s. More recently there has been a move towards early excision of burned tissue to remove necrotic tissue. However, this has not reduced fatalities, in burns of large extent, as much as was hoped. A.B. Wallace of Edinburgh, disillusioned by the infection occurring under occlusive dressings, reintroduced the exposure method of burn wound care in 1949. In the USA this was taken up by, amongst others, Edwin Pulaski and

Curtis Artz of the Brooke Army Medical Centre, Texas.

The last 20 years have seen a continuing interest in finding the best topical agent to use to suppress wound infection. The upsurge of antibiotics in the 1960s offered only short-term benefit for burn victims, organisms proving their adaptability by developing resistance to one agent after another. Only the haemolytic *Streptococcus*, once the scourge of burns units, has lessened in importance. But with the advent of the silver compounds, silver nitrate, sulphadiazine and sulphamylon some progress has been achieved in reducing the amount of wound infection.

Publicity via the media and education to prevent burn accidents must remain the priority if much suffering is to be avoided.

References

COCKSHOTT, W. P.(1956) The History of the Treatment of Burns. *Surg. Gynaec. Obstet.*, 102, 116.

EVANS, E. I., PURNELL, O. J., ROBINETTE, P. W., BATCHELOR, A. & MARTIN, M. (1952) Fluid and Electrolyte Requirements in Severe Burns. *Ann. Surg.*, 135, 804.

HAUBEN, D. J., YANAI, E. & MAHLER, D.(1981) History of the Treatment of Burns. *Burns*, **7**, 383.

MONAFO, M. W.(1971) *The Treatment of Burns*. W. H. Green Inc., St. Louis, Missouri.

SCARBOROUGH, J.(1980) Medications for Burns in Classical Antiquity. *Clin. Plastic Surg.*, **10**, 603.

THOMSEN, M.(1977) Historical Landmarks in the Treatment of Burns. *Br. J. Plastic Surg.*, **30**, 212.

WAKELEY, C. P. G.(1940) War Burns. In Hamilton Baily (ed.). *Surgery of Modern Warfare*. E. and S. Livingstone, Edinburgh.

WALLACE, A. B.(1949) Treatment of Burns: Return to Basic Principles. *Br. J. Plastic Surg.*, **1**, 232.

WALLACE, A. F.(1982) *The Progress of Plastic Surgery*. W. A. Meeus, Oxford.

2

Aetiology, Incidence, Mortality and Prevention

In the United Kingdom about 900 deaths a year occur as a result of injury by fire. It has been calculated that each year 150 000 people attend British accident departments with burn injuries, of which 15 000 are admitted to hospital. In the USA, 300 000 people are hospitalized each year of which 60 000 are children, and 7000 die.

Table 2.1 Incidence of burn patients in a large European city

	Number (per thousand population per annum)
Number of burned inpatients	0.3
Likely deaths	0.01
Number of outpatients treated	2.9
Treated by GPs	0.8
Total burned patients	4.1
Average length of inpatient stay	20.5 days

Table 2.2 Age distribution of burn injuries

Age group	Incidence of age group in population (%)	Incidence of burn injury as % of all burn injuries
Less than 5 yrs	6	23
5–15 yrs	11	10
16–59 yrs	62	61
Over 60 yrs	21	6

Source: Sorensen and Thomsen (1969) *Panminerva Medica*, **11**, 1–2.

In making arrangements in clinics and hospitals for care of burned patients, the incidences as experienced in a large European city are helpful (Table 2.1). The type of injury varies according to the rural or industrial nature of the environment, the predominant type of heating in the homes etc., but in many reports the age distribution remains surprisingly constant (Table 2.2). Clearly, children are

4

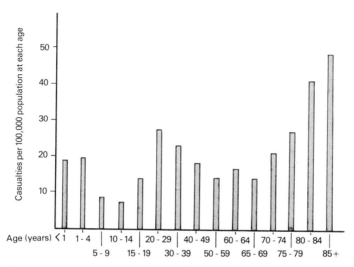

Fig. 2.1 Fire burn casualties per 100 000 population by age

particularly at risk, but the great majority of these injuries are scalds, frequently less deep and extensive than fire burns. When fire injuries alone are considered, young adults and the elderly over 70 years are especially prone (Fig. 2.1).

Deaths from burning (903 in 1983 in the United Kingdom) are most common in the elderly. After the age of 70 years, the mortality rises rapidly, but very young children are more at risk than their older counterparts with an equivalent size of burn (Fig. 2.2).

The majority of fire casualties occur in houses (7137 (65%) non-fatal per annum, and 710 (6%) fatal). To this must be added the hospitalized scald injuries to children, perhaps another 7000, which occur almost exclusively in homes. Only 18% of non-fatal and 10% of fatal fire injuries occur in other buildings such as factories, hotels, schools and restaurants (Fig. 2.3).

Cooking appliances left on or unattended are responsible for starting 35% of all home fires and account for 27% of non-fatal and 6% of fatal casualties. More devastating still are cigarettes, cigars, pipe ash and matches, which are responsible for 28% of non-fatal and 39% of fatal casualties. Heating appliances such as electric and gas fires and heaters lead to 13% of non-fatal and 19% of fatal casualties.

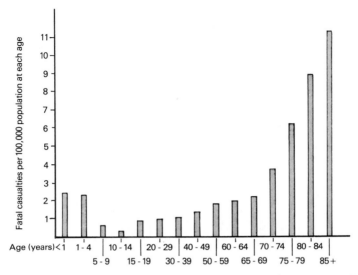

Fig. 2.2   Fatal fire casualties per 100 000 population by age (From *Fire Statistics, United Kingdom.* Home Office, 1983)

Types of Burn Injury

The five main types of burn injury are:

1 *Scalds*: Injury from hot fluids, tea, coffee, bath water. These are often partial thickness.
2 *Flame*: Ignition of clothing from unguarded gas and electric fires, open coal fires, explosion of paraffin and petrol ignited bonfires. In the elderly, a cigarette dropped into the armchair or bedclothes is all too often fatal. Burning fat in chip pans also produces deep burns. *Flash* burns occur when skin is momentarily exposed to high temperature.
3 *Chemical*: In military conflicts, napalm and phosphorus. Bleaches, domestic cleansers, industrial acids and alkalis, agricultural lime. Cytotoxic drugs injected extravenously by accident can produce extensive tissue necrosis.
4 *Electrical*: High tension overhead or underground power cables carry 32 000 volts or more. Contact with the cable may be accompanied by violent propulsion of the patient in the explosion, causing fractures or intraperitoneal bleeding. Domestic burns (240 volts a.c.) occur when a live terminal or wire is touched, while the

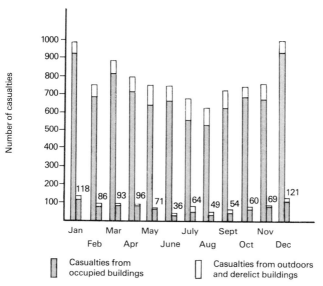

Fig. 2.3   Fire casualties by month. The first of each pair of columns represents the number of non-fatal casualties and the second the fatal casualties. (From *Fire Statistics, United Kingdom*. Home Office, 1983)

patient is earthed, sometimes with his feet in water (as when leaning out of the bath to operate a faulty light switch).

5 *Radiation*: Burns from inadvertent escape of nuclear fuels, accidents during radiotherapy or deliberate use of destructive weapons. The wound is slow to heal because of the induced thrombo-angiitis, and the resultant scar tissue is prone to repeated ulceration.

Of the above, scald and flame injury are responsible for 75% of burns, the remainder the other 25%.

Inhalation Burns

The great importance of the adverse effect on survival of inhalation of hot gases or smoke is shown in Table 2.3. Out of 903 fatal fire casualties, 61% had inhaled gas or smoke, although inhalation burns constituted only 21% of the casualties.

Table 2.3   Casualties recovered from fires

	Fatal casualties	% of all fatalities	Non-fatal casualties	% of all fire casualties
Burned	249	28	3093	28
Overcome by gas or smoke	553	61	1710	16
Physical injury			561	5
'Shock' only			1373	12
Unspecified and precautionary check–up	101	11	3483	32
Total	903	100	10 043	93

Source: Fire Statistics, U.K., 1983.

Mortality

The death or survival of the burned patient depends chiefly on:
  his age. The very young and the old are particularly prone to death
  from the complications of burn injury;
  the amount of the body surface burned.

Table 2.4 shows that, in statistical terms 100 patients aged up to 14
years with a burn of less than 32% body surface area would all be
expected to survive. Of 100 patients aged 50 years with a burn of
30% body surface area, 20 would be expected to die. For any
individual, however, there are factors which influence the outcome
predicted from such figures. These tables help only to assess results
in retrospect, when a large number of patients has been treated.

Additional factors which may influence the outcome are:
  previous cardiac or respiratory disease, or diabetes mellitus;
  the presence of serious wound contamination and infection;
  the inhalation of noxious gases or smoke.

Prevention

Since 75% of burn accidents in the United Kingdom occur in the
home, publicity about the causes of domestic accidents is likely to
produce the greatest benefits. Such publicity is given through
television and radio, newspapers and magazines. Care in design of
potentially dangerous kitchen and heating equipment, and the

Table 2.4 Statistical values of mortality with age and percentage area of body burned (0.1 = 10% mortality, 0.9 = 90% mortality).

Area of body burned %	0–4	5–14	15–24	25–34	35–44	45–54	55–64	65–74	75+
93+	1	1	1	1	1	1	1	1	1
83–92	0.9	0.9	0.9	0.9	1	1	1	1	1
73–82	0.7	0.8	0.8	0.9	0.9	1	1	1	1
63–72	0.5	0.6	0.6	0.7	0.8	0.9	1	1	1
53–62	0.3	0.3	0.4	0.5	0.7	0.8	0.9	1	1
43–52	0.2	0.2	0.2	0.3	0.5	0.6	0.8	1	1
33–42	0.1	0.1	0.1	0.2	0.3	0.4	0.6	0.9	1
23–32	0	0	0	0.1	0.1	0.2	0.4	0.7	1
13–22	0	0	0	0	0	0.1	0.2	0.4	0.7
3–12	0	0	0	0	0	0	0.1	0.2	0.4
0–2	0	0	0	0	0	0	0	0.1	0.3

(Age (years))

Source: Adapted from Bull, 1971.

imposition of legal standards on the flammability of clothing and upholstery, continue to play a part in reducing injury.

Ten basic domestic precautions:

1 The positioning of hot liquids on shelves or table tops out of reach of the toddler or crawler, and the removal of table cloths which may be dragged off the table bringing dangerous liquids with them;
2 The exclusion of children from the kitchen or bathroom, by gates if necessary;
3 The equipping of all kitchens with fire-resistant cloths or towels;
4 The installation of guard rails round the tops of gas and electric ovens;
5 The fitting of secured fire guards round open fires;
6 The avoidance of trailing electric flexes attached to kettles;
7 Ceiling mounting of electric light switch cords in bathrooms;
8 The locking of domestic bleaches and cleansers away from the reach of children, in safety stoppered bottles;
9 Prohibition of smoking in bed in old people's homes or hospitals;
10 The fitting of domestic electrical sockets with safety cut-out.

References

BERRY, C. C., WACHTEL, T. L. & FRANK, H. A.(1982) Analysis of Factors which Predict Burn Mortality. *Burns,* **9**, 38.

BOSS, W. K. & ARONS, M. S.(1982) Molten Metal Safety Boot Burns. *J. Trauma,* **22**, 884.

BULL, J. P.(1971) Revised Analysis of Mortality due to Burns. *Lancet,* **ii**, 1133.

BYROM, R. R., WORD, E. L. *et al.* (1984) Epidemiology of Flame Burn Injuries. *Burns,* **11**, 1.

CARVAJAL, H. F. & PARKS, D. H.(1982) Survival Statistics in Burned Patients. *J. Burn Care Rehab.,* **3**, 81.

FELLER, I., JAMES, M. H. & JONES, C. A.(1982) Burn Epidemiology. *J. Burn Care Rehab.,* **3**, 285.

Fire Statistics, United Kingdom. (1983) Home Office.

GLASHEEN, W. P., ATTINGER, E. O., ANNE, A.*et al.* (1982) Identification of the High-risk Population for Serious Burn Injuries. *Burns,* **9**, 193.

GLASHEEN, W. P., ATTINGER, E. O., ANNE, A. *et al.* (1982) Epidemiology of Minor Burn Injuries. *Burns,* **8**, 423.

GRIFFITHS, R. W. & LAING, J. E.(1981) Burn Injury in the Aged Patient. *Burns,* **7**, 365.

LANARES, A. Z. & LINARES, H. A.(1980) Burn Prevention Programmes for Children. *Burns,* **6**, 73.

LINARES, H. A.(1981) 115 Consecutive Autopsies in Burned Children. *Burns,* **8**, 263.

MURDOCK, R. & EVA, J.(1974) Home Accidents to Children Under 15 years: Survey of 910 cases. *Br. Med. J.,* **2**, 103.

OLLSTEIN, R. N.(1982) Burn Prevention. *J. Burn Care Rehab.,* **3**, 267.

PEGG, S. P., MCDONALD, G. P., PATTE, C. E. T. & MAYZE, T. D.(1983) Epidemiology of Burns Attending a Casualty Department in Brisbane. *Burns,* **9**, 416.

PEGG, S. P. & SEAWRIGHT, A. A.(1983) Burns due to Cooking Oils. *Burns,* **9**, 362.

PRUITT, B. A., TUMBUSCH, W. T., MASON, A. D. & PEARSON, E. (1964) Mortality in 1100 Consecutive Burns Treated at a Burns Unit. *Ann. Surg.,* **159**, 396.

PURDUE, G. F., HUNT, J. L.*et al.* (1985) Burns in Motor Accidents. *J. Trauma,* **25**, 216.

ROSENBERG, B., STERNBERG, N., ZAGHER, U.*et al.* (1982) Burns due to Terrorist Attacks. *Burns,* **9**, 21.

RYAN, R. F. & RASMUSSEN, J. E.(1968) Burns in Children. *Plastic Recon. Surg.,* **42**, 334.

SORENSEN, B. AND THOMSEN, M.(1969) Total Number and Economic Consequences of Burn Injuries in a Scandinavian Population. *Panminerva Med.,* **11**, 51.

SORENSEN, B. & THOMSEN, M.(1980) Cost of Burn Injuries in Denmark. *Burns,* **7**, 162.

YIACOUMETTIS, A.(1976) An Analysis of Burns in Children. *Burns,* **3**, 195.

YOSHIOKA, T., OHASHI, Y., SUGIMOTO, H. *et al.* (1982) Epidemiological Analysis of Deaths from Burns in Japan. *Burns,* **8**, 414.

3

Skin and Pathophysiology of the Burn

Skin

Anatomy

An adult has about $1.8\,m^2$ of skin; it is one of the largest organs in the body (see p.53).

Skin consists of:

1 An outer layer of epidermis (Fig. 3.1), comprising a basement layer of cells which divide and are shed towards the surface, gradually becoming flatter. The cells lose their nuclei to become the dead horny keratin surface layer. A cell migrates from basement membrane to keratin layer in about 19 days. On areas such as the soles of the feet, this keratin layer is thick so that the skin is often protected from deep burning.

2 A inner layer of dermis consisting of collagen and elastic fibres, nerve endings and blood vessels. Deep in this layer are the sweat glands, sebaceous glands and hair follicles, which are derived from the epidermis, growing down into it during embryonic development. Thick dermis, such as occurs on the back, may also protect against full-thickness burning.

Beneath the dermis is a plexus of capillaries and the subdermal layer of fat.

Function of Skin

1 Heat regulation:
   (a) Dilatation or constriction of the dermal and subdermal vessels permits more or less blood to the body surface. Heat is lost from the surface by radiation provided the air temperature is below surface body temperature.

11

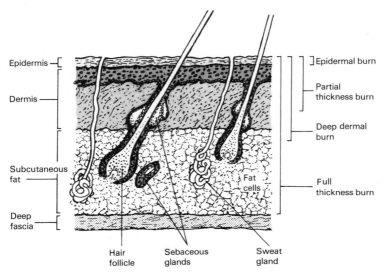

Fig. 3.1   Histology of skin

(b) Evaporation of sweat uses energy, in the form of heat. When sweat is discharged onto the skin surface and evaporates, the skin surface is cooled. Dilation of the vessels to bring more blood to the skin therefore increases the loss of heat (see p. 14).

2 Protection from bacterial invasion. Once vesels in the dermis are exposed by burning or ulceration, bacteria, yeasts and viruses colonize and penetrate the wound.

3 Maintenance of fluid and protein within the body. Intact keratin is nearly waterproof whereas dermis denuded of epidermis is permeable. Except via glandular secretion, little or no fluid, protein or electrolytes pass through intact skin.

4 Control of electrolyte balance. Copious sweating causes loss of sodium and chloride ions as well as of water.

5 Protection from solar radiation. Melanocytes in the basement layer of skin react to ultraviolet by the production of melanin pigment which absorbs ultraviolet rays.

6 Production of Vitamin D.

7 Sensibility to the environment, via nerve endings in the dermis.

8 Determination of the individual's characteristic appearance.

Burn injury to the skin deranges these functions and causes the following pathophysiological changes (see Table 3.1):

1 When damage is small, such as in a light sunburn, capillaries in the dermis become widely dilated, resulting in redness. Some fluid loss from the capillaries into the tissues may cause a rise in interstitial tissue pressure, stimulation of nerve endings and pain.

2 In a more severe burn, the fluid loss from the capillaries accumulates into blisters, either within the dermis or at the junction of dermis with epidermis. The overlying epidermal cells die and are regenerated from adjacent epithelium.

3 When a burn destroys the upper part of the dermis in addition to epidermis, regeneration occurs from the deeper layers of the dermis and from epithelial elements in the glands and hair follicles. Healing of such **partial thickness burns** is complete within 10–14 days.

4 More severe injury destroys the dermis leaving a few epithelial remnants in glands and hair follicles only in the subdermal fat layer. This **deep dermal burn** may re-epithelialize slowly with poor thin skin, and should therefore be treated as a **full thickness burn**.

5 Destruction of all skin elements, a **full thickness burn** may also burn underlying muscle, bone or tendon. This burn requires skin grafting or skin flap cover.

Table 3.1 Clinical depth of burn

	History	*Appearance*	*Blisters*	*Sensation*	*Result*
Superficial	Momentary exposure or sunburn	Red, bloated	Absent	Painful	Heals 7 days
Partial thickness	Scalds of limited duration	Red or pink with a capillary return	Present or surface wet or waxy	Painful	Heals 14 days
Full thickness	Contact with high temperatures. Chemicals. Electrical injury	Charred, brown or white, dry thrombosed vessels	Absent	Painless	Granulates

Circulation Changes and Fluid Loss

Immediately after burn injury, the skin circulation ceases, mainly because of thrombosis in vessels. In a partial thickness burn the circulation is restored within 12–36 hours, but avascularity persists in a full thickness burn until the dead tissue is removed and granulation occurs.

Throughout the body, and away from the burned area, in the case of the more extensive burns, permeability of the capillaries to the lower-molecular-weight proteins, such as albumin, increases. The electron microscope shows that the cells in the capillary walls become rounded instead of elliptical, so developing gaps between them. The cause of this phenomenon is unclear but seems to be due to changes in the globulin fraction of the plasma proteins.

The passage of albumin, electrolytes and water into the extra-vascular tissue space from the capillaries rapidly leads to hypo-volaemic shock, which occurs within a few hours of the burn injury. This effect is exacerbated by increasing amounts of albumin in the tissues which raise the tissue osmotic pressure, and attract water out of the circulation. Fortunately, these fluid changes are usually short-lived and much of the capillary wall integrity is regained within 48 hours of injury (see p.35).

Heat Loss

Large quantities of heat are lost from the burned patient due to:
1 loss of the thermoregulatory function of damaged skin;
2 increased evaporation of fluid from the weeping burn.

Under normal conditions in a climate of 20°C and 40% relative humidity, an adult produces about 290 kJ/h (70 kcal). This pro-duction is balanced by energy loss due to combination of evapora-tion, radiation, convection and conduction, the first two being the chief methods of heat disposal.

The evaporation of 100 ml of water consumes 210 kJ (50 kcals) which drains heat energy from the body. Under the abnormal condi-tions of additional water loss in a burned patient, heat loss may ex-ceed body heat production, unless additional energy is supplied in the form of a high ambient room temperature (up to 28°C or more), additional radiation warmth, and additional calories from nutrition (see p.159).

For a burned child up to 12 years, the nutritional requirement is shown in Table 19.1. For burned adults, the daily nutritional requirements may be calculated from the formulae:

Calories: 80 kJ (19 kcal) per kg body weight + 300 kJ (72 kcal) for each 1% body surface burned.
Protein: 1 g per kg body weight + 3g for each 1% surface area burned.

Red Cells

Red blood cells undergo changes after burn injury. There is an immediate haemolysis in the region of the burn, but additionally red cells have a reduced life span so that the haemoglobin level may fall markedly within a few days of injury. Because the responsible factor seems to be in the plasma of the patient, any transfused blood undergoes the same haemolysis as the patient's own cells. For this reason, it is preferable to give transfusion, if needed, a few days after injury rather than within the first few hours. Despite a reduction in the number of circulating red cells, the haemoconcentration may mask an anaemia if measured by the haemoglobin level.

With the loss of water from capillaries into the tissues, red blood cells become concentrated in the circulation (raised haematocrit). Because of the increased concentration of cells and raised blood viscosity within the capillaries the blood flow becomes impeded and tissue anoxia follows.

The Heart

Following major burn injury, cardiac output falls within half an hour or so to a third of normal. This initial fall is obligatory and is unaffected by prompt transfusion. However, transfusion to replace circulating fluid volume, can prevent or reduce a *later* fall in cardiac output from 6 to 8 hours post-injury.

The initial fall appears to be due to release of a circulating plasma factor, possibly angiotensin, while the later fall results from a reduced right atrial pressure.

The Kidney

Under the action of angiotensin, renal blood flow and urine output diminish after a severe burn. Sodium is retained and potassium (up to 200 mmol/l/day) is excreted, so that potassium supplements may be required towards the end of the period of fluid replacement.

Acute tubular necrosis may follow inadequate fluid replacement. Release of large quantities of haemoglobin from damaged red cells, or myoglobin from damaged muscle, may block tubules resulting in anuria.

Glycosuria occurs in large stressed burns due to depletion of pancreatic insulin often accompanied by a high carbohydrate diet. This pseudo-diabetes is differentiated from true diabetes by the absence of ketones in the urine and by a glucose tolerance test.

Protein Balance

In the healthy body, protein synthesis and breakdown are in equilibrium. In the burned patient, synthesis is usually normal but breakdown is greatly accelerated. This can be measured by urine urea and creatinine estimations, and continues until the skin wound is healed.

The catabolic state is expressed in terms of weight loss which can be remedied by high protein, high calorie diets. More than 10% loss from the initial (admission) weight indicates serious and often irreversible metabolic changes.

Gastro-intestinal Tract

The early vomiting often experienced when forcing oral fluids into the recent burned victim is the result of gastric dilatation and intestinal ileus due to splanchnic vasoconstriction. A nasogastric tube may be passed to empty the stomach if this is troublesome, and fluid intake by mouth or tube reduced to a volume the patient can tolerate. It is usually possible to increase the fluid intake again after the first 24 hours.

When vomiting commences after the resuscitation period it is likely to be a result of severe wound sepsis or septicaemia. Electrolyte imbalance with hypokalaemia is an occasional cause.

Unexplained hypotension, haematemesis or melaena may result from ulceration of the gastro-intestinal tract, usually from multiple points. If the patient has a history of peptic ulceration the bleeding may be seen on endoscopy to be from a single site, but otherwise diffuse bleeding is more common. Blood transfusion is indicated, but the complication is a serious one and the mortality high, indicating the severity of the systemic effect (often sepsis) of the burn injury. Some patients may be saved from continuous bleeding by subtotal gastrectomy. Antacids and H_2 antagonists may be helpful in controlling bleeding.

The Lungs

Lung damage initially occurs from the inhalation of hot air or gas, from irritants such as smoke and from anoxia (see p.125)

The upper airway, nasal passages, mouth, pharynx and trachea respond to injury by oedema leading to obstruction. The bronchioles and alveoli also become oedematous and perfusion becomes inadequate. Acidosis ensues as carbon dioxide is not cleared.

Ventilation is hampered by encircling eschar (burned full thickness skin and dried serum) around the chest, by the outpouring of transudate into the alveolar spaces and by elevation of the diaphragm by intestinal ileus (see p.35). Hyperventilation may therefore result, as an attempt to compensate for the imbalance between ventilation and perfusion.

References

ARTURSON, M. G.(1985) Pathophysiology of Severe Thermal Injury. *J. Burn Care,* **6**, 129.

ARTURSON, M. G.(1978) Metabolic Changes following Thermal Injury. *World J. Surg.,* **2**, 203.

DAVIES, J. W. L.(1982) *Physiological Reactions to Burn Injury.* Academic Press, London.

O'YA, H.(1976) Inhalation Burn. *Burns,* **2**, 115.

SEARCY, R. M., CONE, J. B.*et al.* (1982) High Dose Cimetidine in Acute Thermal Injury. *Burns,* **9**, 62.

SEVITT, S.(1974) *Reactions to Injuries and Burns.* Wm. Heinemann, London.

YAO-LIANG, L. & KE-JIAN, Y.(1983) Prevention of Stress Ulcer Bleeding with Cimetidine in Severe Burns. *Burns,* **9**, 327.

4

First Aid

Prompt and appropriate first aid at the moment of burning and for the first few minutes after the injury may make the difference between a potentially devastating burn and a moderate one, or a moderate burn and a minor one. Few of us will be required to react correctly and quickly at the scene of an injury, but everyone should to be ready to do so if necessary.

In all instances, the patency of the airway must first be assured.

Hot Fluids and Scalds

Spillage of hot fluids or the inadvertent plunging of a limb or a child into very hot water requires:
1 Immediate removal of any soaked clothing;
2 Immersion of the scalded part under cold running water for 5 to 10 minutes. This both relieves the pain and reduces the tissue destruction caused by heat;
3 Drying of the affected part and covering with clean linen (a pillow case or cotton sheet), preferably not fluffy;
4 Removal of constricting rings, bracelets, boots etc. before the part swells;
5 Keeping the patient warm and comforted;
6 Giving small quantities of warm fluids, such as tea, by mouth while waiting for;
7 Rapid transfer to the nearest accident department.

Flame

1 When clothing is alight, the victim should be firmly and gently pushed to the ground, chest downwards. This prevents air reaching the underside of the body and deflects the flames away from the head and face. (Fig. 4.1).

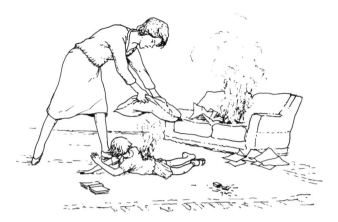

Fig. 4.1 Illustration to show cause of a fire in a room and immediate management to put out flames

2 The flaming clothing is smothered with a cushion, coat, rug, pillowcase, corner of the carpet etc. If those are not available, the patient is slowly rolled on the floor.

3 If the furniture is also on fire, the victim is removed from the room as quickly as possible to prevent inhalation of toxic or hot gases.

4 The hot outer clothes should now be quickly removed and the burned area doused with cold or lukewarm water to remove the residual heat. It is preferable to leave the clothing which has become adherent to the skin, since its removal may pull off potentially viable skin.

5 The victim is dried, kept warm, comforted and given warm drinks, up to 25 ml (quarter of a cupful) every 15 minutes.

6 If pain is severe, a small does of pethidine or morphine may be injected *intravenously*, and the forehead marked with a P or M to alert the casualty officer that analgesia has been given. (Intramuscular injections may not be absorbed due to peripheral vasoconstriction.)

7 The patient is rapidly transferred to the accident department.

Chemical Burns (see p.91)

1 With a few uncommon exceptions, diluting the chemical with copious quantities of water will limit the tissue damage. The water must be delivered quickly in large quantities, i.e. buckets of water

showered over the burn, or from a hose or shower, and repeated for 5–10 minutes.

2 Cover the burned area with a clean sheet or pillowcase.

3 Keep the patient warm with blankets, and transfer rapidly to hospital.

When clothing has been impregnated this is removed quickly, underclothing included.

The Eye (see p.94)

Copious irrigation with water with the patient lying supine. One attendant holds open the eyelids while the other irrigates from the medial side (running the water onto the medial canthic region so that it flows across the globe and drains off the lateral side).

Irrigation is continued for at least 30 minutes (and may be continued at hospital for up to 48 hours with normal saline).

To avoid abrading the cornea, no eye cover is used. Once the irrigation is discontinued, chloramphenicol eye ointment 1% is used 4 hourly.

The ophthalmologist is consulted early and may undertake slit-lamp examination.

Specific Chemicals

Hydrofluoric acid: Massage calcium gluconate gel 2.5% into the burned area (p.92).

Sulphuric acid: Magnesium oxide, lime water or soap are antidotes (p.93).

Alkalis: Vinegar is an antidote (p.93).

Metallic sodium, potassium, lithium: Avoid water application since the mixture is explosive. Smear the surface with grease, or oil. Transfer at once to hospital (p.95).

Bitumen: do not try to remove if it is at all adherent. Convey to the accident department (p.96).

Phosphorus: Keep the skin wet with water-soaked dressings while transferring to hospital (p.95).

Ingestion of Chemicals: Administer large amounts of water to drink. (Milk is an antidote for acid ingestion.) Transfer to hospital at once (p.96).

Cyanide: Where ingestion or inhalation is occurring, remove the source and give 10 ml 3% sodium nitrite IV, 3 ml/min and 50 ml 25% sodium thiosulphate IV, 5 ml/min.

Electrical Burns (see p.83) (Fig. 4.2)

1 The current must first be switched off or the patient disconnected from the supply, using a non-conductor such as a piece of dry wood. NB: when the victim remains in contact with high voltage cables or rails, **no attempt at rescue must be made until the apparatus has been made safe.** High voltages may 'jump' many metres.
2 On verifying cessation of breathing and pulse, external cardiac massage and mouth-to-mouth resuscitation is started (Fixed dilated pupils are not necessarily a sign of irreversible brain damage, particularly with lightning-strike injuries.)
3 Ensure patency of the airway.
4 All electrical burns victims should be admitted to hospital, at least for observation for 24 hours. (If the patient has been thrown by high-tension shock, avoid unnecessary neck movements and apply a temporary neck collar during transportation.)

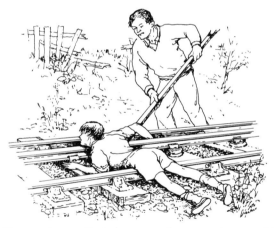

Fig. 4.2 Unconscious patient electrocuted on a conductor rail being rescued with a non-conducting piece of wood or branch

Inhalation Injury (see p.125)

If the patient is rescued unconscious, though breathing, he is turned onto his chest, face to one side, and kept warm with blankets until the ambulance arrives. Any saliva in the mouth may be wiped out with a finger wrapped in a handkerchief. Give mouth-to-mouth resuscitation and cardiac massage as appropriate.

A burn victim rescued from a smoke-filled room or an enclosed space containing hot gases requires immediate oxygen therapy by mask once the patency of the airway has been assured. Oxygen will be available in the ambulance.

Frostbite (Cold Injury)

Destruction of tissue results from:
1 intracellular ice crystals disrupting the cell;
2 ischaemia from vasoconstriction of vessels;
3 intracapillary sludging of hyperviscous blood.

Management

Initial: The patient is withdrawn from the cold environment, wrapped in aluminium foil, 'space-blanket' or thick garments.

Drinking alcohol produces skin vasodilatation, inducing a feeling of warmth but at the expense of further heat loss from the body. Despite St Bernard, it should not be employed! Rubbing the affected part with snow is likely to produce injury to the skin and is also inadvisable.

In hospital: The frostbitten part is rapidly rewarmed in water at 38°C (100°F), dried, elevated and kept at room temperature of about 21°C (70°F).

Heparinization is carried out and an infusion of Dextran 40 to improve the circulation is begun.

Late: When necrotic areas have declared, and before infection supervenes, judicious amputations or debridement are performed. There is no hurry in performing these, and spontaneous separation of dry gangrene often leaves less reconstruction to be carried out than early surgical interference.

Transportation

Whereas emergency ambulance or car transport may be available for transfer to an accident department a few miles away, air transport should be considered when long distances are involved. Within the first 4 hours of injury, provided an appropriate intravenous regime and a nasogastric tube for aspiration in the case of gastric dilatation and ileus have been instituted, burned patients travel well.

Relative contra-indications to air transport include:

1 patients with cardiac failure or pneumonia;
2 patients with untreated cardiac arrhythmias;
3 patients with large blood losses (from other injuries or gastro-intestinal ulceration).

References

BOYKIN, J. V.(1980) Cold Water Treatment of Scald Injury. *Surg. Forum,* **31**, 555.

BOYKIN, J. V. & CRUTE, S. L.(1982) Burn Shock Protection by Cold Water Treatment. *J. Trauma,* **22**, 859.

DAVIES, J. W. L.(1982) Prompt Cooling of Burned Areas; Benefits and the Effector Mechanisms. *Burns,* **9**, 1.

DEMLING, R. H., MAZESS, R. B. & WOLBERG, W.(1979) Effect of Cold Water Immersion on Burn Oedema. *J. Trauma,* **19**, 56.

EDLICH, R. F., SHELLEY, R. *et al.* (1983). Firefighters Guide to Emergency Resuscitation, *J. Burn Care Rehab.,* **4**, 367.

GARDINER, A. W. & FOSTER, S.Teaching Safety, Accident Prevention and First Aid in Schools. *Burns,* **2**, 204.

HARRISON, G. C. & WRIGHT, P. C. (1978) *Medical Management of the Critically Ill.* Academic Press, London.

JONES, M. K.(1984) Fire: Heading off Disaster. *Am. J. Nursing,* **84**, 1368.

KESWANI, M. H.(1977) First Aid and Transport of the Burned Patient. *Burns,* **4**, 46.

LEONARD, L. G., SCHEULEN, J. J. & MUNSTER, A. M.(1982) Chemical Burns: Effect of Prompt First Aid. *J. Trauma,* **22**, 420.

SORENSEN, B.(1967) First Aid in Burn Injuries. *Modern Treatment,* **4**, 1199.

5

Accident and Emergency Department Management

Unless special arrangements have been made, the ambulance service in the United Kingdom usually transports a burns victim to the nearest Accident and Emergency Department.

It is helpful if prior notification of arrival of a major burn casualty is given to the hospital staff by means of radio and telephone links. When a major burn casualty is expected the admitting surgical and anaesthetic resuscitation staff, the sister of the Burns Unit or intensive care ward sister are alerted.

Preparation for Arrival

The resuscitation room prepared to receive the patient must be large enough to accommodate the surgical team, the resuscitation team, a large volume of equipment, and provide sufficient space to permit easy access to the patient from all sides of the casualty stretcher. It may be necessary to use the Accident Department theatre for this purpose.

The room should be well heated (to at least 24°–28°C 75°–80°F), and well ventilated so that body temperature control may be assisted by rapid adjustment of the room temperature.

The equipment specified in the Appendix (p.245) is prepared for use.

Safeguarding the Airway

1 Suction of the nares and mouth is performed if there is respiratory obstruction.
2 If the patient is unconscious, an anaesthetic oral airway is inserted.
3 If cyanosed or the skin is cherry-red (suggesting carbon monoxide poisoning), oxygen is administered by mask (see p.126).

24

4 Endotracheal intubation, preferably through the nose, is necessary if a patent airway cannot be maintained by other means. Endotracheal tubes of latex with low pressure cuffs may be left in place for several days. The cuffs need not be periodically deflated; to do so merely permits debris to slip down the trachea (see p.130).
Tracheostomy should rarely be performed in burns since the direct access of infection into the lungs often outweighs the advantages of easy nursing access to the trachea.
5 Laboured respiration or laryngeal stridor may indicate burning of the larynx or obstruction of the airway by secretion or mucus. If suction and endotracheal intubation fail to relieve the obstruction, bronchoscopy is indicated.

Bleeding

Burn wounds themselves rarely bleed, but blood may be lost from associated injuries. Thus lacerations, fractures or intra-abdominal injury may result in blood loss which requires urgent transfusion replacement.

Analgesia

Full thickness burns are largely painless since nerve endings have been destroyed. Partial thickness burns are extremely painful. In practice most burns are of mixed partial and full thickness. Pain relief may be achieved by patient-administered nitrous oxide and air mixture (Entonox), but morphine may be required. Since a poor peripheral circulation results in non-absorption of drugs from intramuscular or subcutaneous sites, analgesia is given intravenously. Morphine should be avoided in the presence of inhalation or head injury.

Shock

Neurogenic shock: Pain from an extensive superficial burn may be responsible for initiating shock. Morphine is given slowly by intravenous injection. But more usually the cause of shock in burns is **hypovolaemia,** i.e. loss of circulating plasma volume resulting from the transfer of electrolytes, the lower-molecular-weight proteins (abumin) and water into the extravascular tissue space from the circulation. Fluid is also lost from the burned surface which may 'weep' profusely.

History

From the patient, witnesses, ambulance officers and police an accurate account of the accident is obtained. Background information about the patient is obtained from relatives (who may not have been present at the accident) and the family practitioner.

Ten important points to be established:
1 The precise nature of the burn, e.g. scald, electrical, flame, chemical.
2 The circumstances of the injury.
3 The time of the accident (which is the time at which physiological responses to the injury commence).
4 Whether the patient was in an enclosed space (likelihood of inhalation injury).
5 The approximate temperature of the burning or scalding agent.
6 The length of time of exposure to the agent.
7 Details of protective clothing worn.
8 A medical history of pre-existing illness, e.g. diabetes, coronary artery disease.
9 Details of medication already given for the injury, or medication the patient is taking for pre-existing disease.
10 Details of drug intolerance (e.g. penicillin hypersensitivity), or allergies.

Examination and Records

1 The attendant's hair, nose and mouth are covered to prevent contamination of the wound. A clean apron or gown is worn.
2 In preparation for examination, dressings and clothing are removed gently, with scissors if necessary.
3 Snipping up seams of clothing may be preferable to its wholesale removal which may involve further damage to skin. Dressings may require soaking off with sterile saline.
4 Wounds should be handled with sterile instruments in gloved hands.

Pulse

Tachycardia in the burned patient may be due to pain, anxiety or hypovolaemia.

Blood Pressure

Because of limb burns, it may be difficult to apply a cuff and to auscultate. Because of the secretion of vasopressors from the adrenal glands, hypertension or normotension may be present despite the presence of hypovolaemia.

Respiration

Laboured or stridorous respiration may indicate laryngeal burning or obstruction of the airway by sputum, secretions or debris. Circumoral burns, swollen oral or nasal mucosa blackened by soot particles suggest inhalation burning (Fig. 5.1. See also p.127).

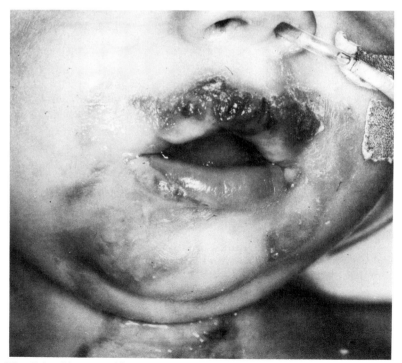

Fig. 5.1 Circumoral burn

Capillary Filling

The state of the peripheral circulation is estimated by lightly pressing on the finger- or toenail, releasing and noting how quickly the blanching of the sub-ungual skin disappears. With a sluggish peripheral circulation, it may take several seconds to return the colour to the skin (Fig. 5.2).

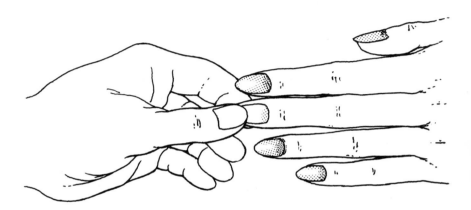

Fig. 5.2   Capillary nail test to show blanching of nail under pressure.

Skin Colour

A cherry-red colour suggests carbon monoxide poisoning. Carbon monoxide has a greater affinity for haemoglobin than oxygen and replaces oxygen in the haemoglobin molecule to form the pink complex, carboxyhaemoglobin (p.126).

Temperature

This is recorded on the temperature chart. Examination of the chest, abdomen, skeletal and neurological systems is undertaken to detect other injury or concomitant disease.

Assessment of the Burn

1 The patient is *weighed* with as few dressings on as is possible. The patient's weight is recorded on the temperature chart.
2 *Surface area;* The extent of the burned surface is a major factor in determining the morbidity and mortality. The relative proportions of different parts of the body (arms, legs, trunk etc.) are shown in Figs 5.3 and 5.4 and vary according to age.

ADULTS:
Exclude areas of erythema from the assessment. Carefully estimate each area burned using the Rule of Nine (see Fig. 5.3). Each of the arms, the head and neck, the chest, the abdomen, the upper back, the lower back and buttocks, each of the thighs, and each of the calves and feet constitute about 9% of the total body skin surface area. For smaller areas of burn, the patient's palm and fingers cover approximately 1% of the body surface.

CHILDREN:
Refer to the 'Lund and Browder' chart (Table 5.1). It shows that the skin surface proportions differ from that of the adult.

Chart the burned areas on an outline of a mannikin in the case notes. Use the convention that areas considered partial thickness burns are singly cross-hatched thus ////, while full thickness burns are double-hatched XXX. Areas of erythema (superficial epidermal burns) are not charted.
Adults with burns exceeding 15% and children with burns exceeding 10% of the total body surface area must be admitted to hospital. Immediate treatment with intravenous fluid replacement is mandatory if they are to survive.

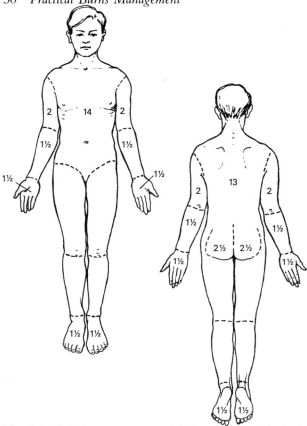

Fig. 5.3   Relative percentages of different parts of the body at all ages

Table 5.1   Relative percentages of different parts of the body at different ages

Age in years	Birth	1	5	10	15	Adult
Head and neck	21%	19%	15%	12%	11%	9%
Thigh	5%	6%	8%	9%	9%	9%
Calf	5%	5%	5%	6%	6%	7%
Foot	3%	3%	3%	3%	3%	3%
Arm	7%	7%	7%	7%	7%	7%
Hand	3%	3%	3%	3%	3%	3%
Chest	7%	7%	7%	7%	7%	7%
Abdomen	7%	7%	7%	7%	7%	7%
Back and buttocks	18%	18%	18%	18%	18%	18%

Source: Modified Lund and Browder

3 *Depth of Burn:* may be clinically
  (a) superficial epidermal
  (b) partial thickness
  (c) full thickness (Fig. 5.5)
  The characteristics of these are shown in Table 5.2. A superficial epidermal burn, exemplified by a sunburn, shows erythema and blistering.
4 *Photography:* While the wound is exposed and undressed, colour photographs are taken to provide an accurate record of the state of the injury.

Table 5.2 Characteristics of burns which when taken together rather than individually may help in the diagnosis of the depth of the burn.

	Partial thickness	*Full thickness*
Length of contact with burning agent	Momentary	More than a few seconds
Temperature of of burning agent	40–55°C	Boiling water or hot metal
Electrical injury	Unlikely	Probable
'Flash' burn without contact	Probable	Possible
Soles of feet and back of trunk	Probable	Possible
Amount of pain in burn	Painful	Painless
Appreciation of sharpness to pin-prick test	'Sharp'	Appreciates touch or anaesthesia
Pressure on burn with forceps	Blanches	No change
Removal of forceps	Circulation returns	No change
Circulation in subcutaneous veins	Present	Absent, thrombosed
Appearance	Pink, blistering	White or charred

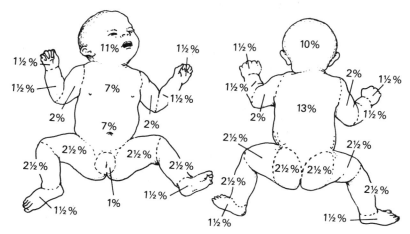

Fig. 5.4   Relative percentages of different parts of the body of a new-born baby

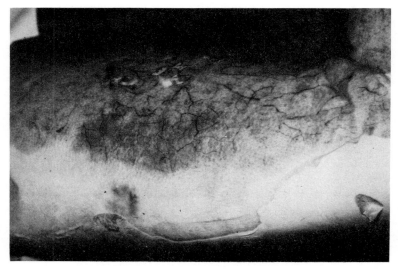

Fig. 5.5   Full thickness burn

Wound cleaning

Bacteriology culture swabs are taken from all burnt areas, mouth, nose and anus. The wound is cleaned with chlorhexidine solution, 0.05%. Dead epithelium and desquamated skin is gently removed with sterile scissors and forceps. Blisters should be punctured; the skin of the roof is allowed to fall back onto the surface to cover the underlying raw epithelium. This acts as a biological dressing conserving fluid and reducing heat loss.

Shaving: Hair harbours bacteria and is therefore clipped to a length of 1–2 cm when it approximates to the burned area. Close shaving should be avoided as this may further damage the skin.

Dressing: A temporary covering of transparent Clingfilm is applied. (Supplied by Bourdon UK Ltd, North Baddersley, Southampton SO5 9ZB or Wrap Film Systems Ltd, Harlesfield 14, Telford, Shropshire TF7 4QR).

Inpatient Management

The following categories of patient require admission to hospital:
1 Adults with burns exceeding 15%, children with burns exceeding 10% and babies with burns exceeding 5% of the body surface.
2 Full thickness burns exceeding 1 in (2.5 cm) in diameter.
3 Full thickness burns of critical areas such as fingers and eyelids.
4 Burns which are circumferential round chest or a limb.
5 Burns of the face, hands, perineum, buttocks or feet.
6 Patients unable to be cared for adequately as out patients.
7 Patients with potentially serious associated medical conditions, e.g. heart disease, other injuries.
8 Electrical burns.
9 Inhalation burns of hot or noxious gas or smoke.
10 Children whose injury is suspected of being non–accidental.

Provided adequate supervision is made, others may be treated on an outpatient basis (see Chapter 6 p.41).

Tetanus toxoid 0.5 ml is given deep subcutaneously if the patient has previous prophylaxis, or human tetanus immunoglobulin (Humotet 250 units) if unprotected.

Laboratory Investigations

Bacteriological swabs are taken from multiple sites of the burn, nose and rectum.

Blood: While the intravenous drip is being inserted, blood is taken for: haemoglobin; haematocrit (packed cell volume); serum electrolytes; blood urea; cross-matching; carboxyhaemoglobin (if carbon monoxide poisoning is suspected); blood gases (if inhalation burn injury is suspected).

Urine: Any urine voided is tested for blood, protein, sugar and 20 ml aliquot kept in a sterile container, labelled with date and time.

Intravenous Fluid Replacement

A reliable fast running intravenous drip is set up, by cut-down if necessary. This latter is particularly necessary in children. The leg is an unsatisfactory site, and the antecubital fossa should be avoided if possible.

Blood for laboratory investigation is taken while setting up the drip (see above). Fluid is infused at a rate which replaces the loss of plasma from the circulation. The initial infusion rate of Human Plasma Protein Fraction is calculated from one of several formulae.

Modified Muir and Barclay Formula

Weight of patient in kg × % surface area burned × ⅔ millilitres is transfused in each of the following periods after the initial burn injury (Fig. 5.6)

Period I	0–4 hours post-burn injury
Period II	4–8 hours post-burn injury
Period III	8–12 hours post-burn injury
Period IV	12–18 hours post-burn injury
Period V	18–24 hours post-burn injury
Period VI	24–36 hours post-burn injury

Plus, for metabolic requirements, oral water:

0–4 years of age	30 ml/hour
5–9 years of age	50 ml/hour
10–14 years of age	75 ml/hour
Adults	100 ml/hour

Thirst may be an early symptom in major burn injury. Oral fluids should be withheld only until the need for intubation and emergency general anaesthesia has been ruled out. When oral fluids are

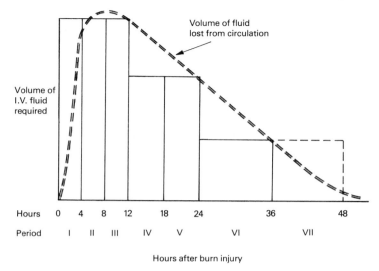

Fig. 5.6 Intravenous fluid replacement following a major burn

commenced it is necessary to restrict the amounts given to those shown in the modified Muir and Barclay formula (above). In patients with severe burns peristalsis may be sluggish or cease altogether (paralytic ileus), therefore excessive oral fluids in the first few hours may provoke vomiting. If oral water cannot be tolerated, an equivalent volume of 5% dextrose is added to the intravenous infusion.

The rate of intravenous infusion is kept as constant as possible throughout the 'period' by:

1 Frequent checks of the drip rate into the drip chamber

Time for 1 litre of fluid to be transfused	*Approximate number of drops per minute*
12 hours	25
8 hours	36
6 hours	50
4 hours	70
2 hours	140

2 This drip rate may be conveniently controlled by using an electronic drip counter or volumetric drip regulator.

3 When administering IV fluids, a burette should be inserted into the line. This is more reliable than counting drops into the drip chamber and allows a check that the fluid is being given at a constant and correct rate.

Escharotomy

Burned skin, when full thickness, contracts. When the whole circumference of an arm, leg, neck or the chest has been burned, the burn therefore acts as a tourniquet, constricting the arteries and veins or, in the case of the neck and chest, the trachea and the expansion of the lungs.

To relieve this constriction, circumferential burns are incised with a sterile scalpel down to bleeding tissue (Fig. 5.7). The procedure is painless since the nerve endings have been destroyed.

Siting of Escharotomies (Fig. 5.8)

While the release of constricting tension may be life- or limb-saving, it will be borne in mind that residual scarring may be worse at the site of a former escharotomy than in other burnt areas. The surgeon sites the incision where it will be most effective in relieving tension and also, if possible, in a site which will leave a concealable scar. The following sites are usually effective, but may have to be varied to meet individual needs:

Chest: A vertical incision 5–7 cm (2–3 inches) lateral to the nipple on each side of the chest.

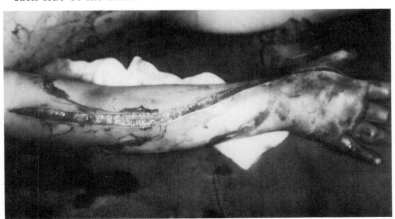

Fig. 5.7   Escharotomy of arm

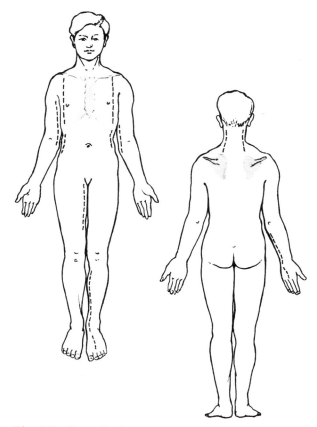

Fig. 5.8 Sites of escharotomy

Neck: Postero-laterally on one or both sides, a vertical incision.

Upper arm: Axially on the medial aspect.

Elbow: Axially on the medial aspect, anterior to the medial epicondyle.

Forearm and wrist: Axially on the medial aspect.

Hand: Axially on the dorsum, between rather than over extensor tendons.

Fingers: Midlateral axial (a unilateral midlateral incision is usually sufficient).

Abdomen: Vertically in both loins.

Thigh: Axially on the medial aspect.

Calf and ankle: Axially on the medial aspect and in front of the medial malleolus.

Foot: On the dorsum between rather than over tendons.

Eyelids

When eyelids have been destroyed, the cornea rapidly dries, leading to corneal ulceration and blindness. Sterile chloramphenicol eye ointment 1% is instilled into the eyes sufficiently often to keep the cornea moist. Eye pads are better avoided as they may produce corneal ulceration by rubbing.

Transfer from the Accident Department

No patient with a major burn remains in the Accident Department for longer than is absolutely necessary to achieve adequate assessment, a reliable intravenous drip running at the appropriate rate and the procedures mentioned above. Speed in transfer for definitive treatment is essential if the patient's morbidity is to be kept to a minimum. Prolonged delays for X-rays, the results of laboratory investigations or the attendance of appropriate staffing militate against the patient's survival.

Whether the patient is transferred to a burns unit or to the intensive care ward of the District General Hospital depends on the extent of the burn, the facilities available at the District Hospital and the availability of beds at the burns unit.

Travel

Most burned patients travel well within the first 4 hours after injury provided adequate resuscitation, including intravenous replacement, and nasogastric intubation have been instituted (see p.50).

Since there may be gross heat loss through burned skin, the patient is kept warm by avoidance of draughts and use of thermal blankets if necessary.

A nurse accompanies the patient and takes with her in the ambulance:

Air and oxygen cylinders
Suction pump and catheters
Anaesthetic mask and airways
Adequate infusion fluids
Ambu bag
Nasogastric tubes
Syringes
Swabs
Analgesia and antiemetic (if prescribed)

All bacteriological swabs and samples (blood and urine) taken from the patient.

If a doctor accompanies the patient, he will also take:

Laryngoscope
Endotracheal tubes and connectors
Drugs for resuscitation
Sterile scalpel and artery forceps

Admission Procedure

Quick Check List for Major Burn

Safeguard airway (see p.24)
History
Full examination, with additional attention to non-burn injuries.
  Chart burns
Patient weighed and recorded
Patient burns photographed
Blood samples for:
  Hb, PCV, WBC
  Serum electrolytes and urea
  Blood group
  Blood gases, carboxyhaemoglobin
IV drip with burette *in situ* with rate of transfusion written up.
Bacteriological swabs from:
  Burned areas
  Nose
  Throat
  Anus
Clean wound and apply temporary dressing
Tetanus prophylaxis given
Escharotomies as necessary
Transfer as quickly as possible to burns unit, intensive care or ward side-room

References

APPS, M. C. P.(1980) Osmolality: Plasma and urine. *B. J. Clin. Equip.* 198.
BAXTER, C. (1979) Fluid Resuscitation, Burn Percentage and Physiologic Age. *J. Trauma,* **19**. Suppl. 11, p.864.
CASON, J. S. (1981) *Treatment of Burns.* Chapman and Hall, London.
FOWLER, J. (1978) Child Maltreatment by Burning. *Burns,* **5**, 83.

KEMBLE, J. V. H. (1983) The Early Management of Burns. *Surgery*, **1**, 52.

KUMAR, P. (1984) Child Abuse by Thermal Injury. *Burns*, **10**, 344.

MAHLER, D. & HAUBEN, D. (1979) Logistic Aids in Treating Massive Burn Casualties. *Burns*, **6**, 146.

MUIR, I. F. K. & BARCLAY, T. L. (1974) *Burns and Their Treatment*. Lloyd-Luke, London.

PRUITT, B. A.(1979) Effectiveness of Fluid Resuscitation. *J. Trauma*, **19**, Suppl. 11, 868.

SETTLE, J. A. (1982) Fluid Therapy in Burns. *J. R. Soc. Med.* **75**, Suppl. 1, 6.

TOWNSEND, P. L. G. (1975) A Cheap and Painless Donor Site Dressing (Clingfilm). *Burns*, **2**, 82.

VURE, E., JOSEPH, M., BEER, S. *et al.* (1981) Burns Shock in Children. *Burns*, **8**, 245.

YING-BEI, Z., YING-JIE, Z. & XUEWEI, W. (1981) Burns during Pregnancy. *Burns*, **8**, 286.

6
Outpatient and Surgery Management

Small burns may be adequately treated on a hospital outpatient basis or by the general practitioner. They include:

1 Partial thickness burns less than about 5% body surface area (see pp.29 and 32).
2 Deep burns (other than electrical burns) less than 2.5 cm (1 inch) diameter on the trunk, arms or legs.

If in doubt, it is preferable to admit the patient and discharge them within a day or two with adequate arrangements for continuing care. The indications for admission of the patient to hospital are given on p.33.

Diagnosis of Burn Depth

Diagnosis of the depth of the burn may be difficult in the first few days but the features in Table 5.2 taken together rather than individually, may be helpful.

General Treatment

1 Adequate analgesia is prescribed.
2 Tetanus prophylaxis is administered.

Wound Management

1 Bacteriological swabs are taken from each burn site.
2 The wound is cleaned with chlorhexidine solution 0.05%.

3 Dead epithelium is carefully snipped away with scissors and metal forceps.
4 Blisters are punctured. It is probably best to allow the blister roof to fall back onto the skin to act as a biological dressing conserving fluid and heat rather than excising it.
5 Hair is clipped when near or in the burned area to facilitate removal of debris and bacteria.
6 The wound is dressed with chlorhexidine tulle gras (one layer), gauze and cotton wool thick enough to prevent seepage of fluid from the burn to the outside of the bandage. For small wounds on the arm Opsite (Smith and Nephew) secured with a crepe bandage is a satisfactory alternative.
7 This is repeated twice weekly until the burn is healed or more often if the dressing becomes soaked.
8 Immobilization and elevation: the burned part is immobilized by suitable dressings or splintage. The patient wears an arm sling, holding the hand up to the shoulder for an arm burn. For a foot or calf burn he elevates the leg on a foot stool during the day when sitting, and raises the foot of the bed by 20 cm (8 in) to encourage drainage at night. By reducing oedema, pain and subsequent scar fibrosis are minimized.
9 Nutrition and fluid intake: because of the metabolic needs involved in healing and the loss of fluid from the burn, a nutritious diet and large oral fluid intake (2.5 litres per 24 hours for an adult and in proportion by body weight for a child) is advised.
10 If the wound is not healed within 14–18 days, it is probable that a full thickness burn has been misdiagnosed as partial thickness. Further time should then not be wasted; skin grafting is undertaken as soon as possible.
11 When the injury is healed, the patient is shown how to apply hydrous ointment (oily cream) three or four times a day, rubbing it well into the scar to soften it.

References

ABSHAGEN, D. (1984) Topical Agents for Minor Burn Injuries. *J. Emergency Nursing,* **10**, 325.
BUCHAN, I.A., ANDREWS, J.K., LANG, S.M. *et al.* (1981) Wound Exudate under Semipermeable Dressings (Opsite). *Burns,* **7**, 326.
WARDEN, G.D., KRAVITZ, M. AND SCHNEBLY, A. (1981) Outpatient Management of Thermal Injuries. *J. Burn Care Rehab,* **2**, 159.

7

Early Care in the District General Hospital

Most patients admitted to the District General Hospital with extensive burns are more satisfactorily managed in a large side room than in the open ward. A side room attached to the intensive care unit is preferable. An ambient temperature of 24°–28°C (75°–80°F) should be attainable. Barrier nursing is strictly observed.

Reassessment of the Burn Injury

One member of the medical staff makes repeated visits to the patient, at least for the first 48 hours after burn injury (see p.48). A senior nurse records and monitors all the patient's signs and symptoms. Key observations are:
General condition of the patient
Respiration rate and quality
Colour of unburnt skin and mucous membranes
Temperature (core and peripheral)
Pulse rate, rhythm and volume
Blood pressure
Urine output, quantity and abnormalities
(Central venous pressure)
(Cardiac function)
(See Chapter 9, p.63)
The doctor responsible for the patient's clinical care *inspects the burn wound* before definitive dressings are applied. He confirms or modifies the accident officer's assessment of the surface area and skin depth burned, and records these accurately on the mannikin in the notes.
In the light of this reassessment, he may modify the volume of fluid to be transfused in the first four-hour period (remembering that if the infusion was not begun until, say, one hour post-burn, he has

43

only the residual 3 hours of the first period to infuse the whole of the first four-hour period's volume) (see p.34).

Wound Cleaning

The wound is cleaned with chlorhexidine 0.05 %. Dead epithelium and desquamated skin is gently removed with sterile iris scissors and metal forceps. Blisters are punctured; the skin of the roof is allowed to fall back onto the surface to cover the underlying raw epithelium. Though not viable this blistered roof acts as a biological dressing reducing fluid and heat loss.

Shaving: Hair harbours bacteria and is therefore clipped to a length of 1 – 2 cm when it approximates or encroaches on burned areas. Closer shaving is avoided as this many further damage the skin.

Dressing or Wound Exposure

The doctor determines what dressing (if any) is to be used (see p.68).
1 If the patient is not to be nursed in a separate room, the wounds will be dressed with:
   A layer of Bactigras tulle
   3 layers of cotton gauze
   2 thick layers of cotton wool
   Crepe bandage
2 If isolation facilities are available, preferably with bacteriologically filtered air, using gloved hands and a wooden spatula, lightly cover the wound with:
   Silver sulphadiazine cream or
   Apply a layer of Bactigras tulle
   Sterile conforming (e.g Kling) bandage

Before the wounds are covered, the doctor satisfies himself that circumferential burns casuing distal ischaemia or venous obstruction have had an adequate escharotomy (see p.36).

A fine-bore naso-gastric feeding tube is inserted.

The bladder is catheterized with a Foley catheter under fully aseptic conditions and allowed free drainage into a measuring closed-system bag, for all patients to whom intravenous fluid is being given. For others, accurate urine output measurements are maintained when the patient passes urine; 20 ml of each sample is retained in a sterile container.

A record is kept of:
  1 colour (see p.144 and Fig. 7.1)
  2 pH
  3 Specific gravity
  4 Protein content
  5 Sugar content
  6 Ketone content
  7 Blood content

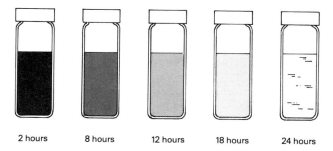

2 hours   8 hours   12 hours   18 hours   24 hours

Fig. 7.1   Serial urine samples showing haemoglobinuria clearing after 24 h

Intravenous Fluids

After the completion of each period, (see p.34) the patient's fluid requirement for the next period is assessed by:
1 Estimation of the hamatocrit (packed cell volume). Deficit (or excess) ml =

$$\text{Blood volume} - \frac{\text{Blood volume} \times \text{normal PCV}}{\text{observed PCV}}$$

Any deficit (or excess) of infusion is corrected in the next period, by adding (or subtracting) this volume to the Muir and Barclay formula prediction for the next period.
2 The urine output, Normal urine outputs are:

  0–1   years of age: 10–20 ml/hour
  1–10 years of age: 20–30 ml/hour
  10–15 years of age: 25–35 ml/hour
  Adults: 35–60 ml/hour

Overinfusion produces urine outputs in excess of the upper limit; underinfusion produces outputs less than the lower limit.

3 The state of the peripheral circulation, pulse rate and volume.

4 The rationality of the patient, lack of restlessness, thirst and sweating.

Thus for period II (from 4 to 8 hours post-burn) the volume of human plasma protein fraction (HPPF) is calculated from the Muir and Barclay formula (see p.34). This is corrected by supplementing or decreasing the formula-predicted volume by the reponse of the haematocrit, urine output and clinical condition of the patient, as determined at the end of the first 4-hour period.

Example: Male aged 16 years.
        Weight of patient 60 kg
        Percentage surface burned 20%
Formula-predicted volume of HPPF required: $60 \times 20 \times \frac{2}{3} = 800$ ml
  Blood volume deficit (or excess) =

$$\text{Normal blood volume} - \frac{\text{Normal blood volume} \times \text{normal PCV}}{\text{Observed PCV}}$$

Patient's normal blood volume (p.238)   5000 ml
        Normal PCV   44
        Observed PCV   50

Blood volume deficit $= 5000 - \dfrac{5000 \times 44}{50} =$ 600 ml

Volume to be infused in second 4 hour period   1400 ml

The same calculation is performed at the end of each subsequent period to determine the volume of HPPF to be infused in the succeeding period. Fig. 7.2 shows how the chart will look. (Note that the formula-predicted volume of 800 ml to be given in the first 4-hour period is given at the rate of 270 ml per hour, since the drip was started one hour into the first period, leaving only 3 hours to the end of this period.)

At the end of period V, the haemoglobin and serum electrolytes are re-estimated. Potassium losses may have been significant; if they need correction, electrolyte supplements are given during period VI and blood transfusion after the end of period VI.

Provided urine output and oral intake are satisfactory, the intravenous drip and urine catheter are removed at the end of period VI. Delaying removal of the IV line increases the likelihood of introducing septicaemia.

RESUSCITATION IV FLUID REGIME

Name..Record No.........................Age..*16*......

Area of burn.....*20%*.....Weight...*60 kg*...Date and time of burn....*1/10/85.* *1am*....

Drip started at...*2:0*.....am/pm on......*1/10/85*...

	Type of Fluid	Volume to be given per hour
1st PERIOD 0 - 4 hours From: *0100* hours To: *0500* PCV *45* %	IV: *HPPF* ORAL *Water*	*270 ml* *100 ml* Signed *A.Doctor.*
2nd PERIOD 4 - 8 hours From: *0500* hours To: *0900* PCV *50* %	IV: *HPPF* ORAL *Water*	*350 ml* *100 ml.* Signed *A.Doctor*
3rd PERIOD 8 - 12 hours From: hours To: PCV %	IV: ORAL	 Signed
4th PERIOD 12 - 18 hours From: hours To: PCV %	IV: ORAL	 Signed
5th PERIOD 18 - 24 hours From: hours To: PCV %	IV: ORAL	 Signed
6th PERIOD 24 - 36 hours From: hours To: PCV %	IV: ORAL	 Signed

Fig. 7.2 Fluid resuscitation chart

Blood Transfusion

Apart from later correction of anaemia, blood transfusion will be required for full thickness burns of more than 20% body surface. The amount of blood given should be 1% of patient's normal blood volume for each 1% area of full thickness burn and is usually given at the end of the 6th period. Transfusion of blood before the end of the 6th period may be necessary but has the following serious drawbacks:

1 The PCV can no longer be used as a reliable measure of calculating the amount of HPPF needed.
2 The transfused red cells are rapidly haemolysed, releasing haemoglobin.

When blood is given before the 6th period, the volume of blood transfused replaces an equal volume of HPPF in the second or third period.

Blood replacement:

Volume of blood to be transfused =

$$\frac{\text{Hb rise required (g\%)} \times \text{blood volume}}{\text{Hb of transfused blood}}$$

(i.e. whole blood 12 g%; packed cells 20 g%)

Rate of intravenous infusion (standard drip set):

ml/h	ml/24 h	drops/min (approx.)
5	120	1.67
42	1000	14
100	2400	33

Table 7.1 gives a summary of fluid management for an uncomplicated burn.

Continuing Reassessment

At the end of each 4 hours, or more frequently if the patient's condition requires, the patient's clinical condition, the charts and the laboratory results are reappraised. This may involve re-examination of the patient's cardiac, respiratory and neurological systems, the abdomen and the limbs. The examination detailed on p.27 is carefully repeated, taking particular note of changes which have occurred since the last examination.

Table 7.1   Summary of IV management for an uncomplicated burn

1st Period 0–4 h	Use fluid formula to determine volume of IV fluid to be infused	
2nd Period 4–8 h	Apply correction to formula volume based on	1 calculated fluid deficit or excess from haematocrit estimated at 4 h post-burn 2 adequacy of hourly urine output 3 condition of patient (e.g. pulse, BP, skin turgor, capillary filling)
3rd Period 8–12 h	Apply correction to formula volume based on	1 2 } as above. Haematocrit 3 } estimated at 8 h post-burn
4th Period 12–18 h	Apply correction to formula volume based on	1 adequacy of hourly urine output 2 condition of patient
5th Period 18–24 h	Apply correction to formula volume based on	1 calculated fluid deficit or excess from haematocrit estimated at 18 h post-burn 2 adequacy of hourly urine output 3 condition of patient
6th Period 24–36 h	Apply correction to formula volume based on	1 adequacy of hourly urine output 2 condition of patient
7th Period 36–48 h (In burns of less than 20% body surface, IV fluids may be discontinued at 36 h. Check electrolytes and haemoglobin before doing so.)	Apply correction to formula volume based on	1 calculated fluid deficit or excess from haematocrit estimated at 36 h post-burn 2 adequacy of hourly urine output 3 condition of patient
	Give blood in place of plasma if burn is greater than 20% body surface, or if patient is anaemic (Hb less than 10.5 g/dl) Correct electrolytes (especially potassium)	Electrolytes estimated at 36 h post-burn

Pulse

A rising pulse rate may indicate inadequate fluid replacement, unsuspected intra-abdominal bleeding, inadequate analgesia or inadequate oxygenation.

Peripheral Circulation

Are escharotomies and fasciotomies sufficient? Causes of cool pale extremities are determined and corrected.

Respiration

A rising respiration rate, stridor and moist inspiration sounds prompt blood gas analysis, laryngeal suction and oxygen therapy. The physiotherapist is alerted.

Abdomen

If there is paralytic ileus and the water being given by mouth or nasogastric tube is not being absorbed, a similar volume of 5% dextrose is given intravenously, and oral feeding temporarily discontinued and the stomach decompressed by aspiration.

Urine

Every hour the catheter bag is emptied. A 20 ml aliquot is kept in sterile container (Fig. 7.1). Record is kept of (a) colour (p.66). (b) pH, (c) specific gravity, (d) protein, (e) sugar, (f) ketone, (g) blood, (h) total volume.

Laboratory Results

Changes in values are often of greater significance than absolute values. It is useful to enter the results on a 'flow-chart' for ease of comparison, without having to refer to several different documents. Most intensive care units already employ such charts which may be easily adapted for the burned patient.

The desirability for one doctor personally to co-ordinate the management of the resuscitation of a patient with a large burn can be readily appreciated when it is recognized that small but rapid changes may indicate progressive deterioration. These may be relatively easy to correct if appropriate action is taken early.

References

ARORA, S. & ANTIA, N.H.(1977) Burns in a District Hospital. *Burns*, **4**, 49.

ARTZ, C.P., MONCRIEF, J.A. & PRUITT, B.A.(1979) *Burns – a Team Approach.* W.B. Saunders, Philadelphia.

DEMLING, R.H.(1983) Improved Survival After Massive Burns. *J. Trauma*, **23**, 179.

JACKSON, D.M. (1953) Diagnosis of the Depth of Burning. *Br. J. Surg.,* **40**, 588.

JONES, R.J., ROE, E.A. & GUPTA, J.L.(1980) Controlled Trial of Pseudomonas Immuno-globulin and Vaccine in Burned Patients. *Lancet*, **ii**, 1263.

MAHLER, D., BARUCHIN, A., HAUBEN, D.*et al.* (1982) Resuscitation of the Burned Patient. *Burns*, **9**, 30.

PEGG, S.P. & SEAWRIGHT, A.A.(1983) Burns Due to Cooking Oils. *Burns*, **9**, 362.

RANGABASHYAN, N.(1977) Early Management of Burns. *Burns*, **4**, 52.

ROE, E.A. & JONES, R.J.(1983) Active and Passive Immunisation against *Pseudomonas aeruginosa. Burns*, **9**, 433.

SAFFLE, J.R., SCHNELBY, A., HOFMANN, A. & WARDEN, G.D.(1983) Management of Fractures in Thermally Injured Patients. *J. Trauma*, **23**, 902.

SETTLE, J.A.D.(1974) *Burns – The first 48 hours.* Smith & Nephew Pharmaceuticals Ltd.

SETTLE, J.A.D.(1974) Urine Output following Severe Burns. *Burns*, **1**, 23.

SUTHERLAND, A.B. Burn Injury – Later Management. *Surgery*, **1**, 423.

VURE, E., JOSEPH, M. *et al.* (1982) Treatment of Burn Shock in Childhood. *Burns*, **8**, 245

WALSH, M.B., MILLER, S.L. & KAGEN, L.T.(1982) Myoglobinuria in Severely Burned Patients. *J. Trauma*, **22**, 6

8

Fluid and Electrolyte Management

Fluid Loss

In large area burns, loss of water from the burned surface may be gross. Partial and full thickness burns lose fluid until the surface eschar becomes hard. In full thickness burns, this loss continues for several weeks and can be reduced by covering the wound with occlusive dressings.

The formula:

(25 + % of body surface burned) × total body surface in square metres

gives a rough estimate of the hourly evaporative loss in millilitres, e.g. a patient with a $1.8\,m^2$ of body surface who has sustained a 40% burn will lose $(25 + 40) \times 1.8 = 117\,ml$ of fluid/hour by evaporation.

This amount should be added to the fluid replaced either by mouth or intravenously for 'metabolic purposes'. (See p.34).

Alternatively, the following formula gives the estimated water loss per 24 hours:

% body surface burned + total body surface area in $cm^2 \times 0.3$

Thus a man with total body surface area of $1.8\,m^2$ $(18\,000\,cm^2)$ with a 40% body surface burn loses

$18\,000 \times 40 \times 0.3 = 2160\,ml$ fluid by evaporation per 24 h

This amount should be given by mouth or added to the intravenous drip as 5% dextrose. For elderly patients with cardiac failure, water supplements will need to be restricted. It will be appreciated that these valuations are approximate only and vary depending (among other factors) on whether the wound is dressed or exposed.

Surface Area Estimation

Body surface area may be calculated from the Figs 8.1 and 8.2. The surface area of patients of varying ages is approximately:

Age (years)	Surface area (m^2)
1	0.45
3	0.56
5	0.70
7	0.85
10	1.10
12	1.28
14	1.36
16	1.53
20	1.70
Adults	1.80

Fig. 8.1   Body surface area normogram (adults). The body surface area may be read off from a ruler across height and weight of patient. (Adapted from Talbot *et al.*, 1952)

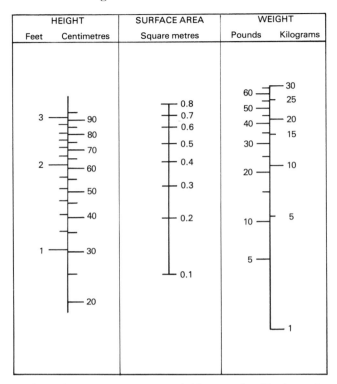

Fig. 8.2   Body surface area normogram (children). Babies' body surface area may be read off by a ruler across height and weight of patient. (Adapted from Talbot *et al.*, 1952)

Water and Electrolyte Depletion

Water Depletion

This follows: Vomiting
                 Diarrhoea
                 Abnormal sweating
                 Haemorrhage
Signs: Dry inelastic skin, dry mouth.
                 Oliguria, urine is concentrated.
                 Low blood pressure and rapid thready pulse.
Symptoms: Intense thirst, confusion, hallucinations.
Serum sodium levels may not be grossly reduced, or may even be normal, in spite of total body depletion.

Sodium depletion

This follows:
  Vomiting
  Diarrhoea
  Abnormal sweating
  Haemorrhage
  Use of diuretics

Signs: Oliguria as the depletion worsens.
           Oedema in extreme cases.
           Clammy, cold, inelastic skin in early period.
Symptoms: Lassitude, anorexia, nausea, vomiting, muscle cramps,
           circulation collapse, convulsions.

Management of Water and Electrolyte Depletion

Calculation of water and electrolyte requirement

Water requirement per 24 hours is the sum of:
1 Basal 24 hour water requirements: for adults, this is calculated by
  insensible loss (sweat, respiration): 500–800 ml (depending on size
  of patient) plus water required for urine formation: 500–1000 ml.
2 The water deficit already present (calculated by previous 24 hour
  intake minus losses from urine, diarrhoea, vomit, gastric aspiration etc.).
3 Estimated additional abnormal water loss during next 24 hours.
  Estimate from the previous 24 hour losses, or, if unknown, add
  1000 ml for moderate diarrhoea or 2000 ml for severe diarrhoea
  and vomiting.
4 Pyrexia. Add 200 ml for each 1°C over 38°C.
  The upper limit should, in almost all cases, not exceed 6 litres per
  24 hours, unless dehydration is gross.

Sodium requirement per 24 hours is calculated from:

  (135 mmol/l minus observed serum sodium concentration) × total
  body fluid in litres.

  Total body fluid is approximately:
  in males: 62% × body weight or 0.62 l/kg body weight
  in females: 52% × body weight or 0.52 l/kg body weight

If the patient is not vomiting and/or has a nasogastric tube the
sodium is most safely given orally:4.5 g of sodium chloride added to
one litre of water (flavoured with fruit juice) and 2 tablespoons (30 g)
of glucose, provides 77 mmol of sodium.

Table 8.1   The amounts of sodium and chloride provided in intravenous solutions

	Sodium (mmol/l)	Chloride (mmol/l)
Normal saline (0.9%)	154	154
⅕ normal saline (0.18%)	31	31
⅗ normal saline (0.54%)	92	92
M/6 sodium lactate	166	0

The amounts of sodium and chloride provided by intravenous solutions are given in Table 8.1. When considering the water and sodium requirements, the number of bottles of different strength solutions are given in approximate proportions. For example, if 4 litres of water and 500 mmol sodium are required to be given in the next 24 hours, alternate litre bottles of normal (0.9%) saline and ⅗ normal (0.54%) saline are given, each in 6 hours.

Hypocalcaemia appearing during the shock phase probably results from calcium binding to injured adipose tissue. Accompanying pancreatitis has been postulated but the evidence for this is at present tenuous. It presents as muscle twitchings and tetany.

Hyperkalaemia may occur early after injury due to release of potassium from injured cells, but is not usually severe enough to need correction provided renal function is normal. To correct hyperkalaemia 20 units of soluble insulin in 30 g glucose or Na^+ resonium 15 g tds orally or PR are given.

Hypokalaemia needs correction at the end of the shock phase when large amounts of potassium have been lost in the urine.

Hypokalaemia

Some degree of hypokalaemia may accompany water and sodium depletion. It also occurs in starvation, profound vomiting and diabetic acidosis.

Symptoms: Muscle fatigue and flaccid paralysis
               Mental disorientation
ECG shows: Flat T waves
               Depressed S–T segment
               Prolonged P–R interval

The potassium deficit is calculated from:

(4 mmol/l minus observed serum potassium level) × total body fluid in litres

Total body fluid is approximately:
    in males   0.62 l/kg body weight
    in females   0.52 l/kg body weight

Since most potassium is intracellular, serum potassium levels may be normal even in the presence of potassium depletion. Therefore the ECG changes (detailed above) should be considered together with the calculated serum potassium deficit.

Potassium replacement

Oral replenishment (preferable to intravenous):
   Potassium chloride tablets 600 mg: each tablet contains 8 mmol of potassium and chloride
   Potassium effervescent (dissolved in water): each tablet contains 6.5 mmol of potassium.
   Bovril: 2 teaspoons in 1 cup of milk contains 14 mmol of potassium.
Intravenous replacement:
   This route should be used only if the hourly urine output is normal,
   Potassium chloride 0.3% and glucose intravenous 5% solution contains 40 mmol of potassium and chloride per litre,
   Potassium chloride 0.3% and sodium chloride 0.9% intravenous solution contains 40 mmol of potassium, 150 mmol of sodium and 190 mmol of chloride per litre.
   A one litre bottle may be infused over 4 hours or more slowly.
   Repeated serum potassium and ECG monitoring is necessary.
   Blood transfusion will raise the serum potassium levels because of the amounts of potassium released from red cells.

Acid–base Equilibrium

In the presence of normal renal function, a reduction of plasma bicarbonate below 22 mmol/l (acidosis) or an increase above 30 mmol/l (alkalosis) will be restored to normal levels by correct rehydration with water and sodium.

However, in such conditions as diabetic coma, salicylate poisoning and renal failure, correction of acidosis with sodium bicarbonate simultaneously with correction of water and sodium depletion is indicated.

Metabolic acidosis often develops within 12–24 hours of injury due to inadequate tissue perfusion and acid release from damaged tissue. Oliguria accompanies a falling arterial pH.

Formula for correction:

MEq of bicarbonate required = base deficit × body weight (kg) × 0.3

If 8.4% sodium bicarbonate is used, 1 mEq = 1 ml. Give in 50 mEq (50 mmol, 50 ml) aliquots over 20 minutes until the full amount has been given. Reassess pH.

Or calculate total plasma bicarbonate deficit by:

(22 mmol/l minus observed serum bicarbonate) × total body fluid in litres.

Total body fluid is approximately:

in males   0.62 litres/kg body weight
in females   0.52 litres/kg body weight

Correction of Acid–base Equilibrium

Intravenous route

Using 1.4% sodium bicarbonate, one litre contains 167 mmol of sodium and bicarbonate. When water and sodium depletion are also present, this may be corrected at the same time using the same considerations as when infusing sodium chloride (page 55).

Oral route

900 mg of sodium bicarbonate powder (given in a flavoured drink) or as tablets (sodium bicarbonate tabs. Co.) provide 12 mmol of sodium and bicarbonate (1 tablet contains 300 mg ≡ 4 mmol).

Alternative IV Replacement Fluids

6% Dextran 70 or 110 in Saline 0.9%

The glucose polymer is a satisfactory and much cheaper substitute for HPPF, but acts only as a plasma expander. It does not replace albumin lost from the circulation. The unmodified Muir and Barclay formula is appropriate to calculate the volume of dextran to be transfused in each period:

wt of patient (kg) × surface area burned × 0.5 (ml)

Ringer's Lactate

The Brook Army Hospital formula uses the following calculation to determine its use:

Plasma 0.5 ml per kilogram body weight per 1% body surface burned

Table 8.2 Fluid contents (per litre bottle)

	Strength (%)	Osmolality	pH	Na^+	K^+	Cl	HCO_3^-	Carbohydrate (g/l)	Protein (g/l)	Calories	Other (mmol)
NaCl (normal)	0.9	308	5.0	150	0	150	0	0	0	0	
Dextrose-saline	4.0	300	4.5	30	0	30	0	40	0	150	
Dextrose 5%	5.0	278	4.0	0	0	0	0	50	0	188	
Ringer lactate (Hartmann's)	5.0	280	6.5	131	5	112	29 (lactate)	0	0	9	Mg 1 Ca 1
Dextran in isotonic saline				144	0	144	0	0	0	0	
Dextran in 5% dextrose				0	0	0	0	50	0	205	
$NaHCO_3$	8.4	2008	8.0	1000	0	0	1000	0	0	0	
$NaHCO_3$	4.2	1004	7.5	500	0	0	500	0	0	0	
Mannitol	10	550									
Ammonium chloride	⅙ M	338		0	0	168	0	0	0	0	NH_4 168
Sodium lactate	⅙ M			167	0	0	167 (lactate)	0	0	0	
Haemaccel	3.5			145	5	145	0			160	Ca 6.25
Plasma		290		152	15	100	0				Ca 2.5
Blood				140	15	103	0				
Packed cells				10	30	26	0				
Human plasma protein				150	2	120			39		

plus Ringer's lactate 1.5 ml/kg body weight per 1% body surface burned
plus 5% glucose to replace insensible losses in 24 hours, half of the total volume to be given in the first 8 hours, and the remaining half in the final 16 hours.

Burns of greater than 50% of body surface are estimated at 50% for the purpose of this formula, so as to avoid overhydration in very extensive burns.

Roehampton Formula

Adults: 120 ml dextran 110 in saline for each 1% body surface burned = total volume of IV fluid required in first 48 hours post-burn, and is divided thus:

½ in first 8 hours
¼ in next 16 hours
¼ in final 24 hours

(Maximum volume to be given is 6 litres)
Plus, for metabolic requirements, oral water, 50 ml/kg body weight per day.
Children:
1   For burns up to 30% of body surface
    the amount of dextran per 1% body surface burned are given in the chart.

	Birth–3 months	3–6 months	6–9 months	9–12 months	1–2 years	2–3 years	3–4 years	4–5 years
Dextran ml per 1% body surface burned	15	21	24	27	30	42	48	54

	5–6 years	6–7 years	7–8 years	8–9 years	9–10 years	10–11 years	11–12 years
Dextran ml per 1% surface burned	63	71	79	87	95	102	111

The figure multiplied by the percentage body surface burned gives the total volume of Dextran required to be transfused over 48 hours, and is divided into
⅓ in first 8 hours

⅓ in next 16 hours
⅓ in final 24 hours
Plus for metabolic requirements, oral water

0–2 years	160 ml/kg body weight per day
2–5 years	100 ml/kg body weight per day
5–8 years	80 ml/kg body weight per day
8–12 years	50 ml/kg body weight per day

2   For burns in excess of 30% body surface area
calculate 10% of body weight in grams.
This figure represents in millilitres the amount of dextran
required to be transfused over 48 hours, and is divided

½ in first 8 hours
¼ in next 16 hours
¼ in final 24 hours

Plus, for metabolic requirements, oral water, as for children with
less than 30% of body surface burned (see above).

Odstock Formula

Weight in kg × 75 millilitres is the estimated volume of fluid to be
infused in 36 hours, and is divided

⅓ in first 8 hours
⅓ in next 12 hours
⅓ in final 16 hours

Plus, for metabolic requirements, up to 120 ml water per hour.

Birmingham Formula

Adults: 1500 ml HPPF per 10% body surface burned in first 24
hours, and divided:

½ in first 8 hours
½ in next 16 hours

Then:
750 ml HPPF per 10% body surface burned in the next 24 hours and
divided:

½ in the next 12 hours
½ in the final 12 hours

Children:1 plasma volume is transfused in the first 24 hours for each
15% body surface burned and half this amount in the next 24 hours.
(1 plasma volume = (100 − haematocrit) × total blood volume)

All these formulae require the predicted volume of fluid to be modified according to the clinical and laboratory responses after each period, or more frequently if necessary.

9

Shock: Nursing, Monitoring and Charting

Any patient with a major burn requires intensive care, frequent reassessment by the doctor and constant surveillance by a qualified nurse, because each patient's response to a major burn injury varies depending on several factors (e.g. pre-trauma fitness). Thus the gravity of the 'burn illness' and effectiveness of treatment is liable to fluctuate. Early detection of such fluctuations and the rapid adjustment of treatment affect the patient's chance of survival (see Chapter 7, p.43).

When monitoring the patient with a major burn injury, the nurse must understand that such trauma does not merely constitute extensive skin destruction. A major burn injury threatens the patient's life in many ways because it affects all the vital systems in the body. It is the nurse's observations and careful charting of small changes in the patient's condition which assist the doctor in evaluating the effectiveness of treatment and estimating the patient's requirements for the next few hours.

On admission, a total assessment by the doctor of all the bodily functions is required to establish the patient's current status and how his body is reacting to the burn injury. This assessment includes:

1 **General impression** of the patient, e.g. very distressed, in pain, agitated, conscious, disorientated, euphoric.
2 **Respiration**, rate and depth of inhalation and effectiveness of expiration. Note any signs of inhalation injury (see p.127), laryngeal stridor, air hunger or bronchospasm, and check symmetry of chest movement.
3 **Colour of skin and mucous membranes**, check unburnt areas for pallor, cyanosis, cherry-red colour.
4 **Temperature**, core and peripheral temperatures.
5 **Pulse**, rate, rhythm and volume of major and peripheral pulses.
6 **Blood pressure**.
7 **Urine output**, measure volume hourly and check for specific gravity, sugar, acetone, albumin and blood. Note colour of urine.

8 **Venous blood** is tested for electrolytes, Hb, PCV.
9 **Arterial blood** is tested for pO_2 and pCO_2.
10 **Weight**.
11 **Pre-existing disease**.
12 **Central venous pressure** (if required).

Following this initial assessment, the nurse continues to monitor frequently, e.g. every half hour, and record her general impression of the patient, his respirations, colour, temperature, pulse and blood pressure. Urine output is measured, and the colour and specific gravity tested, hourly. Additional urine testing for sugar, acetone, albumin and blood is carried out and charted as required.

It is helpful for identifying specific trends and making future assessments if all the above observations are recorded on one chart. Using different colours for each graph facilitates easy reading. Each nurse records her observations in the same style to ensure continuity.

The nurse must understand the importance of reporting to the doctor any significant changes in the patient's condition; therefore she must understand the meaning of what she is observing.

General Impression

Provided personnel caring for the patient are sufficiently experienced, the general impression perceived from the patient's appearance and behaviour is a useful guide to the overall condition of the patient. For example, the early observation of increasing agitation or clouding of consciousness may be the first notable sign of respiratory distress, especially in the young, previously fit adult whose body initially compensates well for any inadequacies.

Respiration

During the shock phase of the burn illness respiratory difficulty may result from:
1 Inhalation of hot or noxious gases which cause:
    irritation of the mucous membranes;
    cough with carbonaceous sputum;
    wheezing and bronchospasm;
    oedema of larynx leading to laryngeal stridor and ultimate airway obstruction;
    pulmonary oedema accompanied by hypoxia;
    hypoxaemia due to carbon monoxide poisoning.

2 Over-correction of hypovolaemia by excessive quantities of intravenous fluids, causing pulmonary oedema.

3 Constriction of the chest and/or abdomen by circumferential eschars, requiring immediate release by escharotomy (see p.36).

4 Other trauma, e.g. rib fractures, pneumothorax or haemothorax.

5 Pre-existing disease, e.g. asthma or bronchitis.

Cyanosis indicates hypoxia which may be due to inefficient exchange of gases at the alveolocapillary membrane or lack of 'free' haemoglobin.

Cherry-red discolouration of the skin denotes carboxyhaemoglobin formation due to carbon monoxide poisoning.

Colour of Skin or Mucous Membranes

Pallor indicates constriction of peripheral blood vessels which may be due to:

hypovolaemia,

pressure on blood vessels from oedema or constriction by eschar,

thrombosis of arteries in electric shock.

Temperature

Since one of the functions of the skin is to control body temperature, extensive skin loss results in defective thermoregulation (see p.11). Any hypothermia or hyperthermia should be corrected so that body energy is conserved, and damage to the heat regulatory centre in the brain is prevented.

Use of an electronic thermometer with a skin probe and a rectal probe, which are retained *in situ* throughout the shock phase, minimizes patient disturbance, saves nursing time and is generally most efficient.

The aim in aiding temperature control is to achieve no more than a 3°C difference between core and peripheral temperature and a core temperature between 39°C and 41°C.

Pulse

In addition to checking central circulation and cardiac function, frequent observation of the peripheral pulses is necessary following burn injury because oedema or constriction due to circumferential eschar may occlude blood vessels, or loss of peripheral pulses may be caused by hypovolaemia.

Urine Output

The urine output is measured hourly on the hour. (For normal anticipated output see p.144.) The colour of the urine is noted. Passing of black urine indicates haemolysis and is an ominous sign, possibly leading to renal failure (see p.144). A low or unaltering specific gravity indicates the kidneys' loss of ability to concentrate the urine (see p.143).

Central Venous Pressure

The central venous pressure indicates the efficiency of the right side of the heart and is sometimes used to determine the adequacy of intravenous fluid replacement. However, it does not give a true picture of circulatory status because it does not take into account the pumping action of both sides of the heart or the vascular tone.

Cyanosis indicates hypoxia which may be due to inefficient exchange of gasses at the alveolocapillary membrane or lack of 'free' haemoglobin.

10

Infection and Wound Management

Since infection of the burn wound and its sequelae are responsible for the majority of fatalities after burn injury, treatment is directed from the outset towards preventing or minimizing the colonization of the wound with organisms.

Burn wounds become infected from:

1 *Physical contact*: Attendants' hands, clothing or dressing material may convey organisms onto the wound. Burn wounds should only be touched with sterilized instruments held in gloved hands with all the sterile precautions that would be taken with a surgical wound.

2 *Other patients*: Infection may be transferred by air or by attendants or by fomites. The number of organisms counted in the air of a dressing room is much reduced when the air is changed by ventilation systems.

3 *Fomites*: Ward baths, bed linen and bed pans may permit the transfer of infection from one patient to another. Baths should be chemically sterilized after each use and lined with disposable polythene sheeting. Bed pans are individual, not communal.

4 *Air*: Organisms are carried on dust particles or water droplets. Pathogens may drop from the attendant's hair or from his nose or mouth onto the exposed wound. Attendants who have *Streptococcus haemolyticus* in their weekly nose and throat swabs are assigned to other duties, and those with *Staphylococcus aureus* treated with chlorhexidine and neomycin (Naseptin).

5 *Insects*: Flies and similar carriers alighting on open wounds may be the source of contamination. This is rare in the United Kingdom, but more common in warmer climes.

6 *Auto-infection*: Many people carry *Staph. aureus* and *Strep. pyogenes* in their throats and noses without symptoms. Similarly *Pseudomonas pyocyanea (aeruginosa)*, *Enterobacter*, *E. coli* and *Strep. faecalis* may be cultured as commensals from the colon and rectum. When these invade the burn wound they become pathogenic in the burned patient who is immunologically deficient.

Whether recently burned skin has been sterilized by the heat or still harbours organisms in the deeper recesses of the sweat and sebaceous glands and hair follicles is contentious. It seems unlikely that recent full-thickness burn wounds would still harbour skin organisms. Studies have failed to show that full-thickness skin biopsies of surgically sterilized skin will grow organisms in culture.

Any dead tissue provides an excellent medium for bacteria to multiply. Therefore frequent debridement of the wound, until all necrotic tissue has been removed, is an important aspect of preventing or minimizing infection.

Wound Care

Initial Cleaning

1 Culture swabs are taken from multiple sites of the burn.
2 The burn is gently cleaned with chlorhexidine solution (0.05%).
3 Dead epithelium is snipped with sterile iris scissors and removed. Blisters are evacuated by puncturing their summit and allowing the dome skin to fall back onto the floor of the blister to act as a biological dressing. Such debridement, done gently and efficiently to remove dead tissue, may take up to an hour.

After initial cleaning, a choice exists as to whether the wound is dressed or covered lightly with an antiseptic and left open to the air. Whereas exposure allows the wound to dry, thus reducing the favourable conditions for growth of organisms, epithelium migrates more rapidly in a moist environment such as is present under a dressing.

Relative indications for use of dressings:
1 Patient is being nursed in an open ward.
2 Outpatient treatment.
3 Gross sepsis.

Relative indications for exposure:
1 Areas difficult to dress, e.g. the face, ears, perineum.
2 Isolation of patient is possible.

Occlusive Dressings

Dressings should be thick enough to exclude ingress of organisms from the environment. Once they become soaked through, they are no longer impermeable and require either replacement or further external padding.

Occlusive dressings have severe drawbacks. They are costly in nursing time, frequently involve repeated imposition of pain to the patient when they are changed, and, by maintaining a warm moist environment, encourage the multiplication of organisms. However, occlusive dressings may be the method of choice if a patient is nursed alongside other patients or has a wound which is small enough to permit outpatient management.

The dressing consists of a single inner layer of Bactigras vaseline gauze, covered with cotton gauze and several layers of cotton wool, bandaged firmly with conforming bandages. Bactigras contains chlorhexidine which has been shown to reduce the colonization of *Staphylococcus aureus* and is effective for up to 7 days.

Exposed Wound

When the patient can be barrier-nursed effectively, and preferably the ambient air rendered bacteriologically sterile, the wound may be left without dressings. This has considerable advantages in reducing the ordeal of dressing changes and saving nursing time. The surface of the partial thickness burn should be kept moist (but not soggy) to encourage re-epithelialization and this can be achieved by the application of a topical antiseptic (see below).

The ambient temperature of the room needs to be kept high (25–28° C, 77–82° F) to minimize body heat loss.

The bed linen requires frequent changing, particularly in the early stages when the wound is leaking large quantities of fluid. When the wound is circumferential, ideally the patient is nursed on an air-fluidized bed or turned every two hours.

Each day the wound is cleaned with saline and necrotic tissue gently removed with scissors and forceps. No-touch technique, masks and proper hair-covering must be practised to avoid contamination of the wound by the attendant.

Partial-thickness burns

The eschar begins to separate spontaneously after about 10–14 days. The loose dead tissue is lifted off with forceps and scissors. Epithelium will have regenerated under the eschar (Fig. 10.1).

Full-thickness burns

Wound care aims at achieving a clean vascularized wound which will accept a skin graft. Frequent wound debridement should be carried out by the nurse and the exposed wound covered with a topical antiseptic.

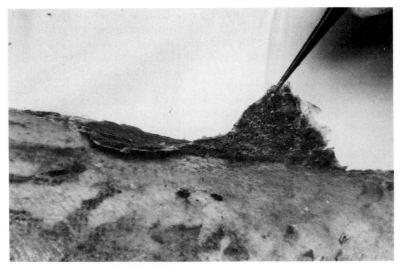

Fig. 10.1   Eschar lifting spontaneously

Difficult Areas to Dress

Face

Even a partial thickness burn of the cheeks, forehead and chin should be admitted to hospital because of the oedema which ensues, often very alarming to patient and relatives. Small areas may be treated exposed, without dressings, and a smear of silver sulphadiazine or chlorhexidine ointment applied. This is renewed daily after saline cleaning of the wound in the outpatient department or surgery.

Hands

Small partial thickness burns of part of the dorsum of the hand or of a digit may be treated without dressings in a polythene bag or large plastic glove (Fig. 10.2). The patient wears a high sling to elevate the hand and is instructed to flex and extend the wrist and fingers fully for five minutes every half hour through the day. At night the hand is raised on four pillows, above the level of the shoulder.

Feet

If the patient can be cared for at home, partial thickness burns of the dorsum of the foot may be treated in a polythene bag, elevating the foot on a foot-stool in the day and on pillows in bed at night.

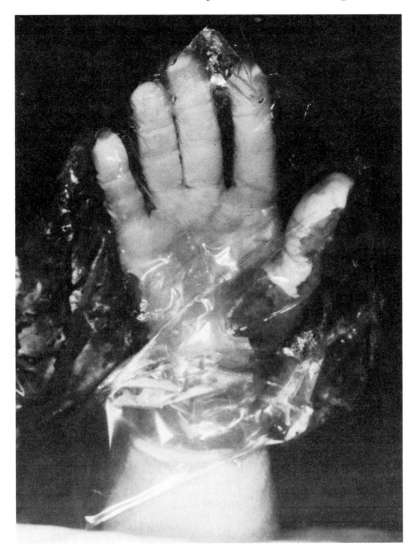

Fig. 10.2 Hand burn in plastic bag

Dressings are, however, often more convenient though elevation is still necessary. The patient should use crutches to move from chair to bed to avoid putting weight on the burned foot.

Ears

Partial thickness burns of the ears are liable to breakdown, exposing cartilage if pressure is applied. Even pressure from lying ear-down on a pillow for a few hours may be sufficient to produce chondritis. When the patient is treated as an outpatient, very generous padding over Bactigras tulle, several layers of fluffed gauze, cotton wool and a lightly applied crepe bandage are used, and the patient instructed to lie on his back.

Circumferential Burns

Burn wounds on which the patient lies become soggy and are difficult to keep clean. Several types of mattress and bed have been tried with varying degrees of success.

Foam mattress★

Thick sheets of polyurethane foam sprayed with silicone aerosol (to minimize sticking) are laid onto an open mesh wire or nylon net-bed frame allowing some gas exchange beneath the patient. Regular turning of the patient is necessary and the foam is discarded as soon as it becomes fouled.

Air-fluidized bed†

The patient is nursed on a sheet covering air–fluidized silicone beads. The air flow helps to dry the wound, and the patient does not have to be turned.

Mediscus low air loss bed‡

Porous sacs inflated with sterile air support the whole length of the patient, thus drying the wound and reducing pressure points.

Antiseptic Topical Applications

Antisepsis is not a substitute for aseptic handling of the wound. Most antiseptic agents are effective only when the organism count is small.
  Chlorhexidine impregnated into vaseline tulle gras ('Bactigras')

★ Supplied by Seton Ltd., Tuberton House, Medlock Street, Oldham, Lancs. OL1 3HS. (Tel: 061 652 2222).
† Supplied by S.S.I. Medical Services Ltd., Finch Close, Lenton Estate, Nottingham, NG7 2NN. (Tel: 0602 866433).
‡ Supplied by Mediscus Products Ltd., Westminster Road, Wareham, Dorset and available for hire. (Tel: 09295 6311).

is particularly effective against staphylococci and provides a useful easy-to-apply dressing. A single layer on the wound is covered with several layers of gauze. It is almost without complications, though very occasionally skin rashes have been reported. Organism resistance has not been reported. Re-application is necessary every 4 or 5 days to maintain its activity.

Silver sulphadiazine 1% The silver salt and the sulphonamide act synergistically. It is mainly effective against Gram-negative organisms such as *Pseudomonas, Klebsiella* and *Escherichia.* The cream is applied with gloved hands not less than every 24 hours, after which it becomes ineffective. Before each application, the wound is cleaned with normal saline. A few *Pseudomonas* organisms are now becoming resistant.

Skin rashes occur and blood levels show that it is absorbed from the wound, rarely giving rise to neutropenia.

The wound becomes soggy when in contact with silver sulphadiazine and this may delay separation of the eschar of a partial thickness burn. The soggy wound is more difficult to debride surgically than the dry wound.

Silver sulphadiazine may be incorporated into a polythene bag in which a burned hand is treated and helps to maintain a moist environment in which the hand may be exercised.

Sulphamylon (Mafenide acetate) 10% as a cream applied twice daily penetrates well into avascular necrotic tissue. It is absorbed as an acid salt, producing a diuresis and hyperventilation. Before each application the old cream should be washed off to prevent caking. In many patients, its use is painful and produces rashes.

Silver nitrate solution 0.5% This solution has the advantages of cheapness and a wide spectrum of efficacy. It is bacteriostatic. The burn wound is first cleaned with warm normal saline; necrotic skin is scrupulously removed since the solution will not penetrate through tissue, ointments or creams.

Cotton wide-meshed gauze is applied to the wounds to a thickness of 1.25 cm (½ inch) and bound into place with a cotton bandage (Kling). Warm silver nitrate (at about 27°C (80°F) is soaked onto the gauze. The whole is covered with dry blankets to reduce heat loss. The procedure of soaking must be repeated every 2 hours; the wound is debrided and the gauze changed daily.

The silver nitrate solution is hypotonic and leaches sodium, potassium, calcium and chloride out of the wound. Coma and convulsions have resulted from a failure to appreciate this and make the appropriate replacements thus:

1 Early morning urine samples are estimated for electrolytes on alternate days.

2 While intravenous fluids are being given, sodium chloride infusion is maintained.

3 After the intravenous route has been discontinued sodium chloride tablets (for an adult 40 g/day) and potassium effervescent are taken by mouth.

4 Calcium supplements (for an adult 6 g/day) are taken.

Since the silver is converted into silver chloride, the dressings, floor, walls and blankets soon become blackened. The worst of these stains may be removed with a water wash after application of iodide (which converts the silver chloride into colourless silver iodide).

Phenoxyethanol 2.2% solution is antibacterial agent, particularly effective against *Pseudomonas pyocyanea* (*aeruginosa*).

Acetic acid 1% The alteration of the wound pH from alkaline to acidic reduces growth of *Pseudomonas pyocyanea*. The length of topical activity depends on the amount of infection, but at least daily applications are usually required.

Topical antibiotic agents such as polymixin, neomycin and gentamycin are liable to produce organism resistance and rashes and are best avoided.

Bath Therapy

Immersion of the patient in a bath of warm water assists in soaking off dressings and facilitates movement. However, infection localized to one part of the body is likely to be spread to all other wounds.

Bathing is therefore reserved for the patient who already has widespread wound infection, confirmed by bacteriological culture swab, or carried out under the guidance of the physiotherapist when the wounds are almost healed.

If wounds in excess of about 25% body surface area are open, salt should be added to the water to prevent loss of sodium from the patient. If salt is added to the bath water to create a 0.9% solution (normal saline), the bath is soothing to the burn wound and speeds up the dressing time by facilitating rapid wholesale removal of dressings. Many patients find wound debridement more comfortable when carried out while the wound is immersed in warm saline.

Dressing Room

Exposure of a large burn wound in an open ward is an unacceptable hazard and all such dressings should be carried out in a dressing room, preferably with a sterilized air-conditioning system.

Full aseptic precautions should be taken, touching the wound only with sterilized instruments in gloved hands and with the attendant properly gowned.

Analgesia

When the wound is large or the patient unduly apprehensive analgesia is given an hour before the procedure is started. Much anxiety can be allayed by a full explanation given by the nurse before embarking on the dressing and less pharmacological analgesia is then required. Diazepam, up to 5 mg in a single dose IV or IM, is used for tranquillizing the nervous. Trimeprazine 3 mg/kg orally or IM is useful for children. Entonox administered by the patient himself can be a very helpful analgesic. General anaesthesia or ketamine anaesthesia is occasionally necessary but is to be avoided if possible since it interferes with the dietary intake of the patient. (See p.122).

Partial Thickness Burns

The aim of wound treatment is the minimizing of wound infection to allow rapid spontaneous healing. This should be complete within not more than 14–17 days. Heavy infestation with organisms may convert a partial thickness wound into a full thickness one. Thus, bacteriological swabs are cultured twice weekly.

Gentle wound debridement is carried out sufficiently often to keep the wound clean (perhaps on alternate days or twice weekly depending on the extent of the wounds and their degree of infection).

The procedure may take an hour and requires empathy between attendants and patient. The wound is cleaned with chlorhexidine 0.05% and debrided with scissors, scalpel and metal forceps, manipulated in gloved hands. Since the attendant will find conversation with the patient a helpful bridge, she wears a mask effective in preventing droplets from her nose and mouth contaminating the wound when she talks. Additionally a plastic apron and a cap to cover the attendant's hair protects both her uniform and the patient's wound.

The wound is covered with an antiseptic, and then either left exposed or dressed with gauze, wool and bandages.

Deep and Full-thickness Burns

Radical excision of burned tissue in patients with burns exceeding about 25% of body surface has been discontinued by many experienced burn surgeons because it gives rise to large blood losses, is traumatic and may spread organisms from the surface to deeper planes. In several clinical trials, it has been shown to confer no benefit.

Therefore, surgical excision is confined to not more than about 20–25% of body surface of priority areas. The remainder is treated by repeated (daily) debridement, gently using forceps, scissors and scalpel. Bacteriological swabs are taken from all sites at least twice weekly.

Debridement of the wound can be carried out quite painlessly, without anaesthesia, because the tissue removed is dead and therefore contains no nerve endings. However, pain may be caused if the process of lifting and cutting the slough pulls on healthy surrounding tissue. Nitrous oxide, administered as gas and air (Entonox), is an effective analgesic for this purpose and will help to reduce anxiety.

Considerable patience is needed on the behalf of the attendant and her patient. Distraction such as conversation, the radio or taped music are helpful in accomplishing a procedure that may take up to an hour. Fear of the debridement should be dispelled before it is started; if this cannot be achieved the procedure must be postponed.

Surgical (theatre) excision is performed within the first 7 days on:
1 relatively small (less than 20% body surface area) burns, or
2 where extensive areas of muscle and fat have been destroyed, or
3 on priority areas such as eyelids, hands, face, axillae, and elbows.

Further surgical excision is repeated after 10–14 days when donor sites have healed and are ready for recropping.

Skin Grafts

Wherever possible excised areas should be covered at once with autograft skin and the extent of the excision confined to that which can be so covered. On the occasion where it is necessary to excise areas larger than available donor sites the excised wound is covered with:

recently harvested cadaver skin,
homograft from a live (usually related) donor,
lyophilized (banked) skin or
vaseline gauze impregnated with chlorhexidine (Bactigras).

Those areas of the burn which have not been surgically excised are dressed with Bactigras or silver sulphadiazine cream.

Homografts and Heterografts

The use of homografts (allografts) from live (usually related) donors or cadavers, or of heterografts (xenografts) from other animal species, usually pig, has been advocated in the following cases.

1 As a temporary covering of burn wounds which, after surgical excision or when granulating, are too extensive to be covered with available autograft. About 10–14 days after the first operation, a second cropping of autograft is taken from the now-healed donor sites and used to replace the homo- or heterografts. This is repeated until the entire burned area has been autografted. There is no good evidence that the use of homo- or heterografts in this manner is preferable to the temporary covering of burn wounds with a dressing and topical antiseptic.

2 To reduce excessive fluid and protein loss from the burn wound. Large fluid losses cease from most burn wounds after 2–3 days, but extensive full-thickness burns may continue large losses for several weeks. Although, theoretically, homo- or heterografting should control these, the practice has proved disappointing. However, when the patient is too ill to permit anaesthesia to harvest grafts, application of homo- or heterografts may buy time.

3 To reduce pain in partial thickness burns.

Care of homo- and heterografts

These grafts need to be inspected daily, cleaned gently with chlorhexidine, and displaced or sloughing grafts removed and replaced. Fever may indicate immune rejection of the grafts, in which case all the grafts must be removed.

Heterografts should, in any case, be replaced every 3 days since they do not acquire a blood supply and if left in place longer produce a dirty, often infected, wound.

Freeze-dried cadaver skin (which can be stored in sterile bags for many months) is commercially available. It is non-viable and non-antigenic, acting only as a dressing, but requires the same care as homo- and heterografts (see above).

Homografts do temporarily acquire a blood supply and if left on the wound for longer than 4 or 5 days become adherent to it. Removal then causes bleeding. It is therefore preferable to renew these completely not less than every 5 days.

Care of Skin Grafts

Skin graft survival depends on the graft acquiring an adequate blood supply from the recipient site. This is achieved by:
1 **Imbibition** Fibrin and elastin 'glue' in the recipient site provides initial bonding within a few hours.
2 **Inosculation** By chance, some capillaries in the graft are in contact with capillaries in the recipient site and these vessels allow some exchange or nutrients within 3 days.
3 **Capillary ingrowth** New capillaries grow from the recipient site into the graft providing a stable blood supply within 5 days.

Causes of graft failure

1 Inadequately excised or debrided eschar.
2 Defective blood supply within the recipient site.
3 Displacement of the graft.
   (a) If left exposed the grafted area is immobilized, protected and observed frequently to ensure that the graft is not accidentally dislodged.
   (b) If a dressing is applied it should be totally adherent, e.g. vaseline gauze (one layer), gauze (one layer), a thick layer of good quality cotton wool and a firm conforming bandage. Graft dressings are removed very carefully, using McIndoe forceps and iris scissors, to ensure that the graft is not accidentally displaced.
4 Infection. Infections which cause copious exudate (e.g. *Pseudomonas aeruginosa*) 'float' the graft off the recipient site. *Streptococcus haemolyticus* destroys skin grafts by lysing epithelial cells.

Septicaemia

The rapid onset of mental confusion, disorientation or lethargy in a previously rational patient arouses the suspicion of septicaemia. Gram-positive organisms may produce the classical high intermittent fever, but gram-negative organisms may induce hypothermia or normothermia. A rise in pulse rate, hypotention, oliguria, vomiting or a rigor may be additional features; skin rashes and pertechiae are rarely seen in burned patients.

Signs which appear late, and are often the prelude to a fatal outcome are oliguria, jaundice and intravascular coagulopathy with cyanosis or gangrene of digits.

On suspicion, blood cultures, a full blood picture and electrolytes estimation are carried out. Blood, preferably freshly donated, is transfused if there is anaemia.

A broad-spectrum antibiotic is given intravenously. If the wound swabs have recently grown large excesses of one particular organism whose sensitivities have been reported, the appropriate antibiotic is used. After 24 hours when the blood culture organisms and sensitivities are reported, the antibiotic is altered if necessary.

Intravenous fluids of plasma protein are given to correct hypovolaemia.

Toxic Shock

The clinical signs and symptoms of septicaemia may be present without the corroborative evidence of a positive blood culture. These cases may be ascribed to the release of toxins from wound organisms to produce systemic effects. Though adults may also be affected, children seem to be more frequently at risk.

The signs are as for septicaemia, often accompanied by a fall in the white cell count. The responsible organism is often *Staph. aureus.*

Blood transfusion plus large doses of intravenous antibiotics with intravenous fluid (plasma) support has been the most effective therapy. The mortality if high, over 50%, when several signs are present.

The possibility of anaerobic infection lurking in necrotic skin or muscle should be treated by adequate debridement together with appropriate antibiotic therapy.

Both septicaemia and toxic shock may be associated with the sick cell syndrome.

Sick Cell Syndrome

An unsatisfactory response of the patient in the first 48 hours after burning may indicate the onset of progressive mental disorientation, metabolic acidosis and over-breathing. Additional signs are oedema and low serum sodium. This is thought to be due to a change in the membrane characteristics of cells.

The 'sodium pump' fails, with potassium leaving the cells and sodium entering. This is recognized by the ratio of urine sodium/potassium changing from the normal 3:1 to 1:1. Serum levels of these electrolytes may be misleading.

Treatment consists of correcting any blood volume deficit by blood transfusion, and administering a glucose and insulin 'cocktail' to drive potassium back into the cells.

Glucose/insulin regime

Adults: Glucose 300 g with 75 units soluble insulin added, given intravenously over 12 hours, together with potassium 50 mEq/24 hours, or more according to the ECG appearances and (less reliably) serum potassium levels. These are given as:
  To 500 ml bottle of 50% glucose add
    Insulin 60 units
    Potassium chloride 10 mEq
    Heparin 1000 units
  Administer at a rate of 50 ml/hour by rapid flush.

If the intravenous line is wanted for other fluids, this amount may be given over a 5-minute period through a three-way tap, and the other fluid administered for the other 55 minutes of each hour, by switching the tap.

Dosage for children:
  Under 2 years ¼ adult dose
  Under 5 years ½ adult dose
  Under 10 years ¾ adult dose

Table 10.1 Titration of blood glucose against dose of insulin

Blood glucose	Additional amount of insulin to be added to 500 ml bottle of 50% glucose	
Over 180 mg %	12 units ⎫	Increase the amount of insulin every 2 hours by this amount until blood glucose is stable around 150 mg %
Over 280 mg %	20 units ⎭	
Below 120 mg %	Reduce by 20 units	

Monitoring response:
1 Monitor blood glucose level two hourly (Dextrostix with capillary blood).
2 Titrate blood glucose against dose of insulin as shown in Table 10.1.
  If urine estimation of glucose is used, glycosuria of greater than 2% is approximately equivalent to a blood glucose of 200 mg%, but this should be checked by comparing at least one blood glucose level estimation made at the same time as a urine glucose estimation.
3 Monitor serum and urine potassium, and adjust dose of potassium accordingly.

Disseminated Intravascular Coagulation

Often accompanying septicaemic shock, disseminated intravascular coagulation (DIC) results in spontaneous bleeding from the burn wound, haematuria, donor skin sites, and occasionally nose-bleeds, bleeding gums, and gastro-intestinal bleeding. Peripheral cyanosis of toes and fingers may lead to gangrene. There is thrombocytopaenia.

Treatment may be successful by the infusion of freshly donated whole blood or fresh frozen plasma. (See p.118).

Hyperthermia

A rise in body temperature is the normal accompaniment of extensive burn injury and does not necessarily indicate infection. Heat losses through burned skin are large and the patient should be nursed in temperatures of 24°–28°C (75°–80°F) at which level comfort is achieved.

Physiological core temperatures up to 40°C (104°F) do not require treatment if pathological causes have been excluded, but above such levels, especially in children, fits are increasingly likely. Tepid sponging and cold fanning serve only to reduce heat losses through normal skin by causing vasoconstriction and are therefore contraindicated when a lowering of core temperature is required. Assurance of an adequate circulation and tissue perfusion by infusion of plasma, correction of anaemia, raising the ambient temperature and removal of bulky dressings are often effective measures. Chlorpromazine may be used for its effect on the hypothalamic temperature regulating centre.

References

ARNOW, P. M., ALLYN, P. P., NICHOLS, E. M. *et al.* (1982) Control of *Staph. aureus* in a Burn Unit: Role of Nurse Staffing. *J. Trauma,* **22**, 954.

BABB, J. R., BRIDGES, K., JACKSON, D. M.,. LOWBURY, E. J. L. & RICKETTS, C. R. (1977) Topical Chemoprophylaxis: Trials in Silver phosphate, Chlorhexidine, Silver Sulphadiazine and Povidine Iodine Preparations. *Burns,* **3**, 65.

BERRY, R. B. & HACKETT, M. E. J.(1980) A Comparative Evaluation of Biological Dressings. *Burns,* **7**, 84.

CAFFEE, H. H. & BINGHAM, H. G.(1982) Leukopenia and Silver Sulfadiazine. *J. Trauma,* **22**, 586.

DIAMOND, A. W.(1982) Analgesia for Burns Dressing. *J. R. Soc. Med.,* **75**, (Suppl. 1) 33.

FEARN, J., AHMED, S. I. & HASAN, N. U.(1976) Acetic Acid in *Pseudomonas* Wound Infection. *Burns,* **3**, 229.

FOX, C. L.(1968) Silver Sulphadiazine: a New Topical Therapy for *Pseudomonas* in Burns. *Arch. Surg.,* **96**, 184.

FRAME, J. D., EVE, M. D.*et al.* (1985) Toxic Shock Syndrome in Burned Children. *Burns,* **11**, 234.

HAMBRAEUS, A., RANSJO, U.(1977) Clothes-born Infection in a Burns Unit. *Hygiene,* **79**, 193.

HARRIS, N. S., COMPTON, J. B.*et al.* (1975) Fresh, Frozen and Lyophylized Porcine Skin on Burned Patients. *Burns,* **2**, 71.

HINTON, P., ALLISON, S. P., LITTLEJOHN, S. & LLOYD, J.(1971) Insulin and Glucose to Reduce Catabolic Response to Injury in Burned Patients. *Lancet,* **i**, 767.

INMAN, R. J., SNELLING, C. F. T., ROBERTS, F. J. *et al.* (1984) Comparison of Silver Sulphadiazine plus Chlorhexidine and Silver Sulphadiazine as Prophylaxis against Burn Wound Infection. *Burns,* **11**, 35.

JACOBY, F.(1984) Care of the Massive Burn Wound. *Critical Care Quart.,* **7**, 44.

JACKSON, D.(1972) Excision and Closure of the Wound as Applied to Burns. *Proc. R. Soc. Med.,* **65**, 23.

KEMBLE, J. V. H., LAMB, B. E.(1984) *Plastic Surgical and Burns Nursing.* Baillière Tindall, London.

KEMBLE, J. V. H.(1980) Management of the Burn Wound and Sepsis. *Hosp. Update,* **6**, 1057.

KIBBE, E(1984) Burn Pain Management. *Critical Care Quart.,* **7**, 54.

LAMKE, L-O., NILSSON, G. E. & REITHNER, H. L.(1977) The Evaporative Water Loss from Burns. *Burns,* **3**, 159.

LAWRENCE, J. C.(1977) An Experimental and Clinical Evaluation of a Tulle Gras Dressing Medicated with Silver Sulphadiazine. *Burns,* **3**, 186.

LAWRENCE, J. C.(1977) Treatment of Burns with Chlorhexidine. *Burns,* **3**, 239.

LOWBURY, E. J. L.(1972) Prevention and Treatment of Sepsis in Burns. *Proc. R. Soc. Med.,* **65**, 25.

LOWBURY, E. J. L.(1975) Recent Studies in Control of Burn Infection. *Burns,* **2**, 26.

MACMILLAN, B. G.(1975) Burn Wound Sepsis – A 10 Year Experience. *Burns,* **2**, 1.

MACMILLAN, B. G.(1978) Symposium on Burns – Closing the Burn Wound. *Surg. Clin. N. Am.,* **58**, 1205.

MAHLER, D. & HIRSHOWITZ, B.(1975) Xenografts in the Treatment of Burns. *Burns,* **2**, 44.

SEVITT, S.(1979) Complications of Burns. *J. Trauma,* **19**, 358.

SHUCK, J. M.(1975) Use of Heteroplastic Grafts. *Burns,* **2**, 47.

SNELLING, C. F. T.(1981) Evaluation of Povidine Iodine and Silver Sulphadiazine for the Burn Wound. *Burns,* **7**, 143.

THOMAS, D. & WITHINGTON, P. S.(1985) Toxic Shock Syndrome. *Ann. R. Coll. Surg.,* **67**, 156.

THOMAS, S., DAWES, C. E. & HAY, N. P.(1983) Medicated Tulle Dressings. *J. Hosp. Infect.,* **4**, 391.

WHO/ISBI WORKSHOP.(1984) Causes, Diagnosis and Management of Serious Infections in Burns. *Burns,* **11**, 41.

11

Electrical Burns

Pathogenesis of Electrical Injury

Electrical current enters the body at the point of contact, travels along planes and structures of low resistance, and exits through the earth contact.

Only the contact points initially produce visible skin injury (Fig. 11.1). Factors which influence the amount of tissue damage include:

1 Voltage. High tension voltages ionize the air particles and may arc across several metres (making physical contact with the electrified conductor unnecessary for the sustaining of injury). Voltages as small as 45 volts have been fatal.

2 Amperage (current) determines the heat generated: Heat $\propto$ resistance $\times$ amps^2. Ventricular fibrillation has been induced by 100 amps on the heart, and the effect of amperage is related to the length of time for which it is applied.

3 Resistance. In ascending order of resistance (least resistance first) blood vessels, nerve, muscle, skin, tendon, fat, bone provide a pathway for passage of the current. Thrombosis of blood vessels may result in ischaemic or venous gangrene of tissue supplied by those vessels, some distance from the burn injury. Dry skin offers a resistance of about 1 million ohms, whereas moist skin only 35 000 ohms. Skin immersed in water has a resistance of 1000 ohms.

Histology

A central area of charring at the point of electrical contact is surrounded by a zone in which tissues are architecturally recognizable but dead. This zone is surrounded by partial necrosis in which the vessels are either necrosed or with intimal and medial wall damage. Muscle shows coagulation of proteins and damage to the myofibrils.

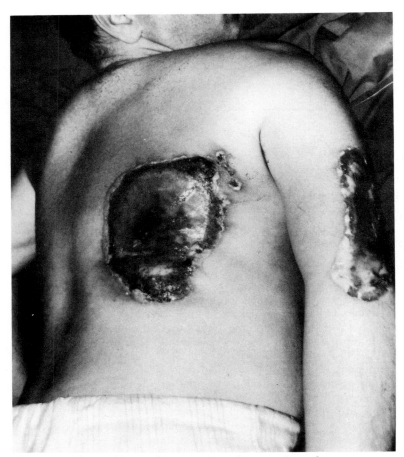

Fig. 11.1   Electrical burns showing exit and entry points of contact

Damage is produced by:
1 Heat caused by passage of the current through tissues.
2 Damage to vessels producing ischaemic necrosis.
3 Interference with electrical conductivity of organs such as the heart and nerves.
4 Tetanic contraction of muscle (particularly with alternating current).
5 Thermal injury from ignition of clothing etc.
6 Forceful propulsion of the body, producing spinal or limb fractures, intraperitoneal and intrathoracic injury.

Physiology

Unexplained hypokalaemia may occur within a few hours of injury and persist for several weeks. This may be explained by alteration of the cell membrane potential caused by the electrical injury affecting electrolyte exchange across the cell wall.

Myoglobin and haemoglobin released into the circulation in large quantities is a measure of the extent of muscle and red cell damage. Unless rapidly excreted, acute renal failure is likely.

Burning by contact with electrical current which passes through the body has effects upon the heart, brain, abdominal cavity, muscle, or blood vessels and nerves. In addition it destroys the skin which comes into contact with the electrical source. For this reason, the estimation of the degree of burning by measuring the skin surface burn is valueless. Considerably greater quantities of tissue may be destroyed beneath intact skin than is superficially apparent.

Alternating current produces greater damage then direct current. Most injuries are caused by the low tension 240 volt alternating domestic supply. Less common injuries occur from high tension electrical supply such as from railway overhead conductors (25 000 volts AC), conductor rails (750 volts DC) or from National Grid electrical cabling (400 000 – 30 000 volts AC)

Low Tension Injuries

Flash Burns

These are caused by momentary exposure of the skin, usually the face and hands, to flash heat without actual contact of the skin to the electrical conductor. Initially the skin looks black, swells (often closing the eyelids alarmingly), and after a few days heals as a partial thickness injury. Such burns are treated by regular cleaning with chlorhexidine, puncturing blisters, and leaving the burn exposed. The hands are elevated to reduce oedema and the fingers mobilized under the guidance of the physiotherapist.

Electric Fire Filament or Electric Bar Burns

These occur usually to the hands, and are almost invariably full thickness. Tendons and nerves may also be destroyed. The main injuring agent is the heat rather than the electrical current. When they occur in children, bone growth potential often seems to be reduced, perhaps because of scar tightness inhibiting bone growth.

These require early (3rd or 4th post-burn day) excision, skin grafting or skin flap cover. Nerves burned but still in continuity should not be divided, as some axonal growth through the burned section may be possible. Similarly tendons burned but still in continuity may be left in place.

Contact with 'Live' Wire

The patient often becomes locked onto the electrical appliance and requires to be disconnected either by turning off the power source or using a non-conductor material. The contact point burn may be only one or two centimetres in diameter, but because of tetanic contraction the victim may be unable to disconnect himself from the source. Hands and mouth (babies chewing wires) are frequent sites. It is important to look for the point of exit of the current from the body, often the soles of the feet.

The wound should be dressed lightly with silver sulphadiazine, or Bactigras tulle, and inspected daily. Dead tissue is excised when the full extent of tissue loss is apparent, usually 10–20 days after injury. Replacement is with skin grafts or flaps. The latter are often preferable since grafts may fail because of poorly vascularized 'electrically damaged' tissues in the bed, but where there are several punctate wounds flaps may be impracticable.

Low tension burns of the hand may be treated conservatively in a polythene bag containing silver sulphadiazine. Active and passive mobilization is pursued. Grafting or flap repair may be undertaken when the extent of the injury is clear.

High Tension Injuries

Physical contact with the wire or cable is not necessary, since the patient may act as conductor in an electrical arc.

Tissue destruction is gross, and may be progressive as initially viable tissue becomes gangrenous due to a microangiopathy causing a deteriorating blood supply.

1 After turning off the electrical supply or disconnecting the patient using a piece of non-conducting material, immediate cardiopulmonary resuscitation for ventricular fibrillation or asystole may be life saving. Other injuries, due to being 'thrown' by the explosion, are not uncommon.

2 Progressive loss of distal circulation or of sensation may indicate the increase in subcutaneous or subfascial oedema occluding

vessels. Urgent relieving escharotomies and/or fasciotomies are required. Dead tissue is excised at the same time.

3 Burns on the abdomen may cause thrombosis of intestinal vessels which leads to intestinal gangrene. Stomach contents are aspirated via a Ryle's tube. Exploratory laparotomy is advisable to detect this before peritonitis ensues.

4 ECG monitoring and estimation of cardiac enzymes (transaminase, creatine phosphokinase) to detect damage to heart muscle is carried out.

5 Dead muscle is debrided to prevent myoglobinuria and gas gangrene. Excisions may have to be repeated on several occasions. amputation may be required, and should be carried out as soon as the extent of the damage is known. Since the hand contains little muscle, early surgical debridement in unnecessary, but relieving fasciotomy and escharotomy (see p.36) may preserve tissue which would otherwise become non-viable.

6 Adequate urine output (see p.66) is maintained by administering intravenous plasma protein fraction and blood. Quantities of 4.5 ml/kg body weight per hour in the first 24 hours to maintain blood volume have been recommended. If haemoglobinuria or myoglobulinuria occur, mannitol (1 g/kg body weight in a 20% solution in 30 minutes, repeated once if no diuresis occurs after 4 hours) is given. Sodium bicarbonate may be necessary to correct acidosis.

7 Lesser degrees of haemolysis detected by 6 or 12 hourly haemoglobin estimations may require blood transfusion in the second 24 hours after injury.

8 Definitive reconstruction should be undertaken only when the full extent of tissue necrosis is known. Since necrosis may be progressive as damaged vessels thrombose, this is rarely practicable before about 2 weeks.

Electric Arc Burns

High tension arcs cause injury by intense heat or flash. The current may earth itself through the victim in contact with the ground, may leap to another nearby object or return to the source.

Cardiac irregularities, or ventricular fibrillation are common. Respiratory failure may occur.

Care of the Electrical Wound

Low tension injuries causing small punctate wounds are dressed with Bactigras tulle or silver sulphadiazine cream. The extent of the tissue necrosis becomes clear after 4–7 days.

The dead tissue is excised and appropriate skin graft or skin flap cover provided.

High tension injuries Early escharotomy and fasciotomy within an hour or two of the injury will probably be required as tissue oedema progresses. Obviously dead muscle should be removed, but it must be borne in mind that further progressive muscle death is likely. Wounds are left open for inspection and assessment for further debridement.

Limbs are elevated and an antiseptic (such as chlorhexidine 0.05%) irrigated or packed lightly into the wound. Frequent re-observation of the wound and limb to assess distal viability is necessary.

Lightning Injuries

Prevention

1 Avoid standing close to potential conductors, (e.g. tall trees, metal umbrellas),
2 If in an open space, squat or crouch, do not stand.
3 Discard some metres away metal golf clubs, fishing rods, etc.

Early Effects

1 Acute myocardial infarction or arrhythmias
2 Muscle necrosis leading to myoglobinuria
3 Coma, seizures and amnesia (cerebral oedema)
4 Paralysis, hyperaesthesia
5 Blast injuries (lung, cerebral haemorrhage, intraperitoneal injury)
6 Burns, of arborescent ('spidery') distribution
7 Gastric and intestinal ileus

Management

1 Cardiopulmonary resuscitation, initially by external cardiac massage, mouth-to-mouth resuscitation and later by endotracheal intubation may be successful even after several hours of apparent

failure. Fixed dilatation of the pupils is not necessarily a sign of irreversible brain death.

2 A central venous pressure line is required to assess the blood volume.

3 Human plasma protein fraction is infused rapidly in amounts sufficient to maintain a urine output in an adult of more than 25 ml/hour (see chart p.66).

4 Mannitol 1 g/kg, sodium bicarbonate and large intravenous fluid volumes are given for metabolic acidosis, haemoglobinuria and myoglobinuria.

5 Continuous stomach aspiration through a Ryle's tube is necessary to prevent pulmonary aspiration of regurgitation due to gastro-intestinal dilatation.

6 Early amputation of limbs with significant muscle damage.

7 Cerebral oedema may respond to dexamethazone and diuretics. Mannitol may lighten coma.

Late Effects

These may include hysteria, hemiplegia, cataract, neuralgia and scar contractures. Although the ECG may initially show an acute infarct pattern this may be replaced by a normal ECG later. It is probable that damaged heart muscle is replaced by scar.

References

BAXTER, C.R.(1970) Present Concepts in the Management of Major Electrical Injury. *Surg. Clinics N. Am.*, **50**, 1401.

BINGHAM, H.G.(1980) Electrical Injuries to the Upper Extremity. *Burns, 7*, 155.

DAVIES, M.R.(1958) Burns caused by electricity. *Br. J. Plastic Surg.*, **11**, 288.

FOGH–ANDERSEN, P. & SORENSEN, B.(1966) Electric Mouth Burns in Children. *Acta Chir. Scand.*, **131**, 214.

HANSON, G.C. & MCILWRAITH, G.R.(1973) Lightning Injury. *Br. Med. J.*, **ii**, 271.

HOUSINGER, T.A. GREEN L.*et al.* (1985) Myocardial Damage in Electrical Injuries. *J. Trauma*, **25**, 122.

LAZARUS, H.M. & HUTTON, W.(1982) Electric Burns & Frostbite. *J. Trauma*, **22**, 581.

MUIR, I.F.K.(1957) Treatment of Electrical Burns. *Br. J. Plastic Surg.*, **10**, 292.

PLAZA, R., QUETGLAS, A. & RODRIGUEZ, E.(1983) Treatment of Electrical Burns of the Mouth. *Burns*, **10**, 49.

ROBSON, M.C., MURPHY, R.C.& HEGGERS, J.P.(1984) Progressive Tissue Loss in Electrical Injuries. *Plastic Recon. Surg.*, **73**, 431.

SAFFLE, J.R. CRANDALL, A. & WARDEN, G.D.(1985) Cataracts. *J. Trauma*, **25**, 17.

SINHA, J.K., KHANNA, N.N., TRIPATHI, F.M.*et al.* (1978) Electrical Burns. *Burns*, **4**, 261.

SKOOG, T.(1970) Electrical Injuries. *J. Trauma,* **10**, 816.

TAUSSIG, H.B.(1968) 'Death' from Lightning and the Possibility of Living Again. *Ann. Intern. Med.,* **68**, 1345.

XUE-WEI, W.(1981) Electrical Burn of the Abdomen with Intestinal Perforation. *Burns,* **8**, 128.

XUE-WEI, W., NAIZE, W., CHANGSHUN, L.*et al.* (1982) Electrical Injury of the Upper Extremities. *Burns,* **9**, 24.

12

Chemical Burns

A very wide variety of chemicals is used in industrial processes. Safety precautions, vigorously pursued, have dramatically reduced the incidence of burn accidents from these sources.

However, domestic accidents continue to occur with unacceptable frequency, and burns deliberately inflicted in time of war from gas, toxic chemicals, incendiary bombs and conflagrations resulting from explosions constitute a significant proportion of the burn casualties.

Some agents (e.g. chromic and formic acids, phenol and organic chemicals) are absorbed through the skin and produce liver and kidney failure, in addition to the local effect on the skin.

The wearing of non-flammable 'anti-flash' gear has been recognized as extremely effective protection in naval conflict ever since the latter years of the 1914–18 World War. The practice again proved its worth in the 1939–45 World War and the Falklands War, 1982.

Industry has learned from the Armed Services by the introduction of compulsory protective clothing, goggles, gaiters, high-ankled boots and long gloves, in those industrial processes where chemicals or flammable liquids are used.

Domestic bleaches and detergents may be made more safe by storage out of reach of children (even when clambering up onto chairs) in 'child-proof' stoppered bottles.

For Poison Advice Centres, see p.255.

Acids

Hydrochloric Acid, Nitric Acid.

The injuries produced are:
1 Local coagulation of skin and subcutaneous tissue, thrombosis of vessels.
2 Absorption into the circulation to cause acidosis (rapid respiration) or renal failure (anuria or high volume of urine with inability to concentrate the urine above specific gravity of 1010)

Immediate treatment

The burned area is washed with copious quantities of running water as quickly after the injury as possible. This is continued for at least several minutes (5–15 min is average), the length of time depending on the extent of the injury and the dose of water being delivered. Smaller quantities of water may worsen the burn by spreading the acid and producing more heat.

At the end of this treatment, sodium bicarbonate 1.4% or a buffer solution of (30 g potassium acid phosphate and 220 gm sodium phosphate dissolved in 1 litre of water and filtered) may be poured onto the burn.

Alternatively soap, magnesium hydroxide or trisilicate or soda lime are effective.

Hydrofluoric Acid

This is now extensively used in chemical plants in the production of high octane fuel. To a lesser extent it is used in glass etching, electroplating, production of insecticides and refrigerants.

It has the following properties:

1 Tissue destruction is progessive extending deeper if the acid is not neutralized adequately.
2 Pain is excessive.
3 The chemical bonds with calcium in the body, thus decreasing serum calcium and leading to tetany, paraesthesiae and cardiac arrest. Oxalic acid also produces hypocalcaemia.

Treatment

The attendant must protect himself from contact (by wearing gloves etc.)

1 Soaked clothing is removed from contact with the patient's skin.
2 The injured part is washed with large quantities of water for several minutes.
3 Massage calcium gluconate gel 2.5% into the skin to relieve the pain and neutralize the acid. This may be continued for 15–20 minutes.
4 For burns in excess of $60 \, cm^2$ ($25 \, in^2$) (about the size of a hand) calcium gluconate tablets, 3.6 g, are given by mouth.
5 Burns of the eye are similarly irrigated with water, and calcium gluconate eye drops instilled.
6 The serum calcium level is estimated, and if low 10% calcium gluconate IV, 10 ml given slowly. This is repeated hourly until the serum calcium remains normal. Hypocalcaemia may be recognized by an ECG tracing of a prolonged Q-T interval.

7 If the acid has penetrated beneath the nails, the nails should be split (under general anaesthesia) to permit adequate access to the subungual skin.

8 Persisting pain or treatment of a hydrofluoric burn more than 30–45 minutes old requires injection of calcium gluconate 10% with hyaluronidase into and around the wound.

9 When the burn pain is not controlled, (indicating continuing deep necrosis), the wound is excised and skin grafted.

Chromic Acid, Tannic Acid, Formic Acid, Picric Acid

Chromic acid may be absorbed to produce liver and renal failure. Ingestion causes peripheral vascular collapse, cramps, coma and glycosuria. Emergency treatment consists of washing with copious water or, if to hand, sodium hyposulphite.

Sulphuric Acid

Since concentrated sulphuric acid reacts exothermically with water to 'explode', water lavage should be avoided, unless the quantity of acid is small and the quantity of water is large.

Magnesium oxide, lime water or soap are more specific antidotes.

Alkalis

Sodium Hydroxide, Potassium Hydroxide, Ammonium Hydroxide, Calcium Oxide (Lime)

The effects of injury are:
1 Local dehydration of tissue, destruction of protein and fat.
2 Absorption to cause metabolic alkalosis (muscle twitching and spasm).

Immediate treatment

The skin is washed with water within a minute or two of the injury. Lime and water (calcium hydroxide) react exothermically, generating heat, so the dry lime is first brushed off and then large quantities of running water are required to remove the remainder.

At the end of 5–15 minutes, ammonium chloride M/6, or acetic acid 1% (vinegar), or the buffer solution (as detailed on page 92) may be run onto the wound.

Since alkalis continue to penetrate into the wound, early excision and skin grafting is preferable.

Sodium Hypochlorite

This is widely used in bleaches, disinfectants and deodorizers. The free chlorine coagulates proteins and swallowing leads to oesophageal strictures. Vomiting, haematemesis, confusion and coma with laryngeal oedema occur.

Milk, eggwhite, milk of magnesia, aluminium hydroxide (but NOT sodium bicarbonate) are given by mouth. In the case of skin contact which is less harmful, the hypochlorite is washed off and the above agents applied topically.

Eyes

Chemical burns with alkalis tend to be deeper and more destructive than with acids, since the alkali reacts with cell lipids and penetrates deeply.

Laboratory staff working with such chemicals should wear protective goggles or spectacles, and emergency first-aid kits for immediate eye irrigation with saline or water showers should be to hand.

The face is immersed in a large bowl of water and the eye opened and closed under water. If this is impossible because of blepharospasm or if the patient is a child, the victim may be laid supine on a table, the head turned to the injured side and the eye kept open with fingers (or, better, a Desmarre retractor) and copiously irrigated with water or saline. Any particulate matter is removed with gauze or cotton wool on an orange stick. Such irrigation is continued for 30 minutes or longer; it takes place at the site of the accident and continues in the ambulance on the way to hospital. Contact lenses are removed so that chemical does not remain trapped in contact with the cornea.

When the chemical has been neutralized, chloramphenicol eye drops 0.5% are instilled every 3 hours. The pupils are dilated with atropine drops 1% every 6 hours to prevent ciliary spasm and synechiae. No bandages are applied so the eye can move freely. This aids drainage and may reduce symblepharon.

The opinion of an ophthalmologist is sought early, before oedema has closed the eyelids making examination difficult. Fluorescein staining to detect corneal damage is feasible only before this occurs.

Metallic Sodium, Potassium and Lithium

These explode and ignite on contact with water. This can have disastrous consequences if it occurs in the skin.

The metal and skin is smeared with grease, KY jelly or oil. The pieces are picked out of the tissue with forceps and placed under oil in a container.

Phosphorus

Phosphorus burns in contact with air. The skin is therefore covered with wet dressings until the phosphorus can be picked out with forceps. When the large pieces have been removed, residual small ones can be identified by darkening the room, and observing phosphorescence. Alternatively, running small amounts of copper sulphate suspension onto the skin converts the phosphorus into copper phosphate which can easily be seen as black particles.

To ensure the conversion of all the phosphorus to less-harmful salts after the identifiable pieces have been picked out, the wound is washed with a suspension of: copper sulphate 2% and sodium bicarbonate 5% in hydroxyethyl cellulose 1%. The copper sulphate is washed off the wound before it is absorbed and causes haemolysis.

If treatment is delayed, phosphorus absorption may result in liver and kidney damage. Early death has occurred with low levels of serum calcium, high levels of serum phosphorus and raised ST segments on the ECG.

Vitamin K should be given.

Organic Chemicals

Petrol, Phenol (Carbolic Acid), Trilene, Cresol (Lysol)

These are absorbed through the skin, and may cause cardiac, respiratory, renal and liver failure, convulsions and coma. Cresol causes methaemoglobinaemia and haemolysis.

Soaked clothing is removed. The skin is wiped dry. Copious amounts of water are used to flush off the residual chemical. A soapy mixture helps to dissolve it. Polyethylene glycol or glycerol are suitable solvents for application after the water treatment. IV fluids (and sodium bicarbonate for carbolic acid burns) may prevent kidney damage. Patients are assured that the dye used in some of the agents colours the skin only temporarily.

Bitumen

Asphalt workers may splash hot bitumen onto the skin. (Fig 12.1). This rapidly sets into a hard wad which adheres to the wound. As re-epithelialization of the skin occurs under this impermeable layer (which is impervious to infection) it separates spontaneously after 10–14 days. When, rarely, it is deemed necessary to remove it (such as when it has glued fingers together), it may be dissolved slowly and with difficulty with paraffin oil or margarine.

Potassium Permanganate

Used in disinfectants, bleaches and deodorizers, potassium permanganate stains the tissues purple and oxidizes to destruction. A thick brown eschar usually results. Copious water to wash off the chemical limits is effect.

Cooking Fat Burns

Increasingly common is the chip pan fat burn. When the fat ignites in the pan, instead of turning off the gas or electricity and capping the pan with a pot lid or plate to exclude air, the anxious cook lifts the pan off the oven and runs towards the door, the flames streaming backwards onto her arm, spilling ignited fat onto her legs.

These burns are usually full-thickness. Although often of small extent, they almost always need excision and grafting, a procedure that is carried out once the circulatory state is stable, usually within a week. Only punctate splash burns less than 2.5 cm (1 inch) can be expected to heal spontaneously without grafting.

Oesophageal Burns

Swallowing of domestic bleaches by children is the main cause of oesophageal burning. Intraoral burns and a history of disappearance of the liquid are strong evidence of ingestion. Large quantities of

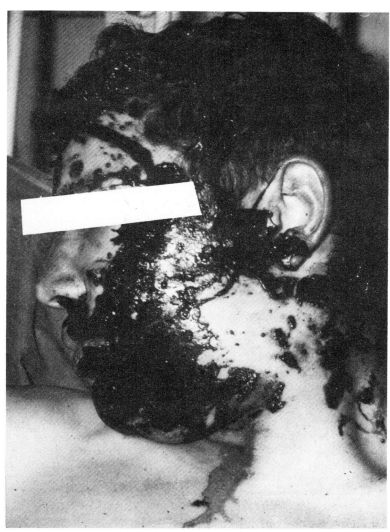

Fig. 12.1 Bitumen burn

fluids are administered by mouth. For acid ingestion, milk is an antidote. Intravenous fluids are given when oral fluids are discontinued, as soon as the initial dilution is complete. Thereafter oral fluids are stopped because of the danger of mediastinal leak.

Oesophagoscopy is diagnostic, but the scope should not be passed into the burned region because of the likelihood of perforation. The chest is X-rayed.

Prednisolone 2 mg/kg/day and ampicillin may be helpful in reducing the swelling and infection. Once bouginage has begun, steriod therapy is discontinued.

A soft or fluid diet is taken when endoscopy indicates that leakage is unlikely. If stricture occurs, bouginage is undertaken, initially under general anaesthetic and later by the patient himself. This is usually reserved until at least the second post-injury week.

Bronchial Burns

Exposure to inhaled gases (e.g. ammonia, methylisocyanate) produces a copious alveolar inflammatory reaction. Steroids and bronchodilators may be helpful. Oxygen, if necessary by endotracheal ventilation, may tide the patient over the period until the oedema subsides (see p.125).

References

ACHAUER, B.M. & MARTINEZ, S.(1984) Tar and Asphalt Burns. *J. Burn Care Rehab.,* **5**, 271

ARWOOD, R., HAMMOND, J. & WARD, G.G.(1985) Ammonia Inhalation. *J. Trauma,* **25**, 444.

ASCH, M.J., MOYLAN, J.A., BRUCK, H.M. & PRUITT, B.A. (1971) Ocular complications Associated with burns. *J. Trauma,* **11**, 857.

BEN-HUR, N. & APPLEBAUM, J. (1975) The Phosphorus Burn and its Specific Treatment. *Burns,* **1**, 222.

GOLDMAN, M. & KAROTIN, R.H.(1965) Acute Pot. bichromate Poisoning. *Am. J. Med. Sci.,* **189**, 400.

HALLER, J.A., ANDREWS, H.G., WHITE, J.J. *et al.* (1971) Pathophysiology and Management of Corrosive Burns of the Oesophagus. *J. Ped. Surg.,* **6**, 578.

HAYASHI, N. (1980) Treatment for Hydrofluoric Acid Burns. *Burns,* **7**, 267.

HUNTER, G.A. (1968) Chemical Burns of the Skin after Contact with Petrol. *Br. J. Plastic Surg.,* **21**, 337.

JELENKO, C. (1974) Chemicals that Burn. *J. Trauma,* **14**, 65.

MATTHEW, H. & LAWSON, A.A.H. (1979) *Treatment of Common Acute Poisonings.* Churchill Livingstone, London.

MOYLAN, J.A., ADIB, K. & BIRNBAUM, M. (1975) Fiberoptic Bronchoscopy following Thermal Injury. *Surg. Gynaec. Obstet.,* **140**, 541.

PARDOE, R., MINAMI, R.T., SATO, M. & SCHLESINGER, S.L. (1976) Phenol Burns. *Burns,* **3**, 29.

PEGG, S.P. & SEAWRIGHT, A.A. (1983) Burns due to Cooking Oils. *Burns,* **9**, 362.

PEGG, S.P. & CAMPBELL, D.C. (1985) Children's Burns due to Cresol. *Burns,* **11**, 294.

PROUDFOOT, A. (1982) *Acute Poisoning.* Blackwell, London.

ROSSIS, C.G. & YIACOUMETTIS, A.M. (1980) Burns caused by Napalm Bombs. *Burns,* **6**, 251.

SCAPA, E. & ESHCHAR, J. (1985) Chemical Burns of the Upper Gastrointestinal Tract. *Burns,* **11**, 269.

SIGURDSSON, J., BJORNSSON, A. & GUDMUNDSSON, S.T. (1983) Formic Acid Burn. *Burns,* **9**, 358.

TEPPERMAN, P.B. (1980) Fatality due to Hydrofluoric Acid Skin Burn. *J. Occup. Med.,* **22**, 691.

VALE, J.A. & MEREDITH, T.J. (1980) Poisoning — Diagnosis and Treatment. Update, London

WALSH, E.N. (1953) Chromate Hazards in Industry. *J. Am. Med. Assoc.,* **153**, 1305

WALTERS, M.J. & LOWELL, G.G. (1982) Corneal Problems in Burned Patients. *J. Burn Care and Rehab.,* **3**, 367.

WANG, X-W., DAVIES, J.W.L., SIRVENT, R.L.Z. & ROBINSON, W.A. (1985) Chromic Acid Burns. *Burns,* **11**, 181.

13

Radiation Burns

Pathogenesis

The electromagnetic spectrum includes radiowaves, infra-red, visible light, ultraviolet, X-rays and gamma rays (in decreasing order of wavelength). All travel at the same speed, and the ability to penetrate living tissue depends on the wavelength and wave frequency. Thus radiowaves and visible light penetrate little or not at all, whereas X-rays and gamma rays penetrate deeply. Repeated exposure accumulates tissue damage.

Onset of apparent effects of injury is shortest with long wavelength radiation, i.e. infra-red 'sunburn', and the longest with gamma rays. Damage at cellular level is to mitosis, enzyme systems and metabolism. Blistering, erythema and swelling of the skin is the minimal reaction, which either returns to normal with little permanent change, or progresses to vessel thrombosis, ulceration and necrosis. Healing by scar tissue is slow and the scar is poorly vascularized. Vitiligo or hyper-pigmentation, telangiectasia, thinning of the epidermis, and malignant scar change are long-term sequelae.

Radiation Overdosage

Following exposure to radiation, such as excessive doses of radiotherapy or radioactive materials and weapons, the tissues undergo a series of changes.

Acute Radiation Syndrome

Depending on the whole-body dosage received the symptoms are:
First Week: Nausea, vomiting and diarrhoea

Headache, disorientation, weakness, erythema, agitation, coma.

Second week: The above plus
Fever, emaciation

Third week: The above plus
Haemorrhage, loss of skin and hair.

Skin Changes

After irradiation, within 24 hours, the skin becomes hot, and reddens. At higher doses, it becomes itchy and is easily abraded if rubbed. Hair loss occurs within two to three weeks. At still higher doses, the skin becomes purple, blisters and ulcerates. At this stage healing is very slow, the scar is avascular, liable to repeated breakdown, and after several years may exhibit malignant change, usually basal or squamous carcinoma, but occasionally sarcoma. Destruction of lymphatics leads to lymphoedema, with recurrent episodes of cellulitis and lymphangitis.

Management

Vomiting and diarrhoea

The loss of fluids and electrolytes from the intestine by vomiting and diarrhoea is corrected by infusion of balanced electrolyte solutions (Hartmann's).

Though of serious prognostic significance, the loss of blood in the diarrhoea is corrected by blood transfusion. Fresh blood is preferable since this contains neutrophils. Neutrophil production decreases in the irradiated patient after the first 48 hours.

Nausea-depressants and appetite stimulants such as pyridoxine, Torecan (10 mg bd) and Stemetil (5 mg bd) may help.

Anti-diarrhoeal agents such as codeine phosphate are given if necessary, but, in the longer term, constipation may ensue due to large bowel fibrosis and lack of peristalsis. Peritoneal adhesions may later produce intestinal obstruction.

The skin

Loss of areas of skin are treated as for a thermal burn with topical antiseptics. Radiotherapists often use gentian violet paint 2% which is fungicidal and bacteriostatic.

Erythematous skin may be washed with lukewarm or cold water, but not with hot water or soap as this would increase the blood supply and the skin reaction. Care is required with shaving; clipping the beard short is preferable to lacerating the delicate skin. The skin is dried by dabbing rather than friction rubbing. A bland talcum powder absorbs moisture and prevents friction.

Dressings are avoided if possible, and generously large clothing of natural fibre such as cotton, or silk is worn, or the erythematous area is left exposed. If a dressing is necessary, it should be light, secured by bandage rather than tape so as not to rub. Zinc oxide strapping increases the skin reaction, but Micropore is suitable if applied and removed carefully. Pressure from bra straps on the shoulders or back, or from spectacles on the face should be avoided when these areas have received radiation damage.

When the erythema has subsided, dry skin may be moistened with aqueous lanolin cream after washing with non-medicated, unperfumed soap.

Unhealed ulcers require flap cover, since their avascularity precludes the successful application of grafts.

Appetite and diet

Exercise, fresh-air and small quantities of alcohol are encouraged as stimulants to appetite. One pint of beer contains 175 calories. Meals are taken regularly and comprise a diet low in residue to spare the bowel. Brown or wholemeal bread, cereals, uncooked green vegetables or fruit, beans, peas, turnips, carrots, plums, and fatty meat are avoided.

Haematuria may occur if the lower abdomen has been irradiated. The patient is encouraged to drink large quantities of fluid to promote urine flow. If clotting causes urethral blockage, catheterization will be necessary, but the catheter is removed at once because of the danger of cystitis.

The eye

Conjunctivitis, or, with larger doses, keratitis is painful and, while initially there may be profuse lacrimation, the secretion later becomes scant and viscid. Dark glasses may be comforting. The lids may be wiped gently with cotton gauze but should not be rubbed. Irrigation of the eye with lukewarm sterile saline allowed to run into the medial canthus is soothing. Albucid drops 10% are bacteriostatic.

Nuclear Explosion

Many burns following nuclear explosion are due to the intense heat-flash, and others from the conflagrations started by the heat. A minority are likely to be due to the radiation itself.

Figures available from the study of the effects of the 12.5 kiloton A-bomb dropped on Hiroshima in 1945, show that almost everyone within 500 metres of ground zero was killed. Of the population within 2 km of ground zero 60% died, three-quarters within the first 24 hours. The deaths occurred mainly from crushing and burning, arising from the initial blast wave followed by the fireball. A typical modern American H-bomb has a power equivalent to 350 kilotons of TNT.

Radiation sickness arises in victims who are exposed to radiation outside the area of blast and fire. Many of these may be from fallout carried downwind.

Anorexia, nausea and vomiting are temporary and reversible.

Bone marrow damage: lymphopaenia occurs within 24 hours, the level giving a good indication of the severity of the exposure. Neutrophils increase for the first 48 hours, and then decrease till about day 10; this is followed by a transient rise at about day 15, which continues to day 30. At about day 30 there is a further fall in neutrophil count, which ceases and begins to rise again after day 35.

Diarrhoea, resulting from failure of mitosis of intestinal wall cells, leads to loss of electrolytes and bacterial infection. Haemorrhagic diarrhoea often precedes septicaemic infections, and death reaches a peak at 30 days falling progressively to about 60 days. The infections can sometimes be controlled with appropriate antibiotics.

Neurovascular syndrome A short interval of alertness is followed by coma.

Skin erythema, and, at higher radiation doses, ulceration, scaling, blistering and hair-loss may recover if the patient survives.

Fertility Sperm production is inhibited and ovulation ceases for periods dependent upon the doses received.

Psychological effects of bereavement, loss, and physical suffering are likely to render the affected population incapable of organized assistance. In the longer term, disabling psychiatric illness is likely to persist for many years in a significant minority of the population.

Triage Whereas non-nuclear mass casualties may be quickly evacuated to nearby hospitals for treatment such facilities are unlikely to be available in a nuclear attack. Since intravenous resuscitation for the thermally injured patient will be unavailable, victims with burns in excess of 25–30% surface area are unlikely to survive in appreciable numbers. Triage, where feasible, will identify (a) those with a poor chance of survival, (b) those with a reasonable chance if treated and (c) those with a good chance with no or postponed treatment.

Self-help and first-aid are the means by which the majority would be managed.

Those with smaller burns should, in ideal circumstances:

1 Drink quantities of uncontaminated water (if available). Since

radiation material tends to fall to the bottom of containers and rivers, running streams should be a safe source, but the surface water from static ponds or lakes should not be used for the first few days.
2 Remain indoors as much as possible to avoid radiation from external fallout for at least 14 days.
3 Arrange for the disposal of urine, faeces and vomit to another part of the building.
4 Maintain a diet of stored food compatible with the (reduced) activity being undertaken bearing in mind future supplies may be limited.

References

BRITISH MEDICAL ASSOCIATION(1983) *The Medical Effects of Nuclear War.* Wiley, Chichester.
COGGLE, J.E.(1983) *Biological Effects of Radiation.* Taylor & Francis, London.
LOCHHEAD, J.N.M.(1983) *Care of the Patient in Radiotherapy.* Blackwell, London.
RÖDING, H.(1981) Ethical Problems in Mass Burn Disasters. *Acta Chir. Plast (Prague),* **23**, 38.
SORENSEN, B.(1979) Mass Casualties after Nuclear Explosion. *Burns,* **6**, 33.
WORLD HEALTH ORGANIZATION(1984) *Effects of Nuclear War on Health and Health Services* (Report of International Committe of Experts). World Health Organization, Geneva.

14

The Burns Operating Theatre

The Timing of Grafting Procedures

Whereas partial thickness burns will heal discarding overlying eschar spontaneously when re-epithelialization has occurred, full-thickness skin loss requires skin grafting, preceded by either surgical excision of the eschar, or repeated debridement in the ward over a period of several days.

If a burn has not re-epithelialized spontaneously within three weeks of the initial injury it is unlikely to do so, and there is little purpose in delaying skin grafting longer (unless the condition of the patient precludes it). The diagnosis of a full-thickness burn should usually have been made long before this time is reached, and appropriate grafting will already have been instituted (see p.32).

First Priority Areas

Where functional contractures should be avoided, e.g. the *hands, across joints* and *eyelids*, granulation tissue should not be allowed to form prior to grafting. Rather, eschar should be excised within a few days of the injury, and the area covered with autograft.

Thus eyelid burns are grafted within 3 days of injury to prevent exposure of the cornea with the possibility of subsequent blindness. Hand burns require grafting within 4 or 5 days to permit the patient, under the physiotherapist's guidance, to commence early mobilization of the wrist and fingers.

Second Priority Areas

Where functional contracture is less important, and some wound contracture may be acceptable, these areas may be treated as regions of lesser priority for grafting by daily repeated wound cleaning and debridement. Such areas are the back, chest and abdomen. Where choices have to be made as to which areas should be grafted first, and which deferred until a subsequent operation, priorities are given to burns in the region of joints, and on the face and neck, where contractures are undesirable.

The timing of removal of eschar and grafting of second priority areas depends upon the following:

1 Is the patient fit enough for anaesthesia?
2 What is the bacteriology of the burn wound? The presence of *Streptococcus haemolyticus*, especially Lancefield group A, precludes grafting, since this destroys new epithelium and grafts.
3 Are there sufficient non-burnt areas of donor autografts to cover the burned areas?

Burns of less than 20% body surface area can often be autografted at a single operation. Unless otherwise indicated this can satisfactorily be undertaken within a week of injury. Burns in excess of 20% body surface area often require two or more operative procedures, separated by a period of 10 to 14 days to permit re-stabilization of the patient and the healing of donor autograft areas from which a second cropping of grafts can then be removed. Thus the first procedure within 7 days of injury is followed by the second procedure at about 17–21 days post-injury.

Escharectomy

Extensive burns in excess of, say, 50% body surface area, require escharectomy in theatre of not more than 20–25% of the body surface at one time; such areas are then covered with autograft. Blood loss is often excessive if areas greater than this have eschar removed at one operation. Un-escharectomized areas are treated daily in the dressing room by debridement gently using scissors and scalpel, day by day removing more and more of the necrotic tissue.

Summary of Grafting for Full-thickness Burns

Graft within 3 days   : Eyelids
Graft within 4–5 days   : Hands, areas of potential tendon
                                or bone exposure
Graft within 7 days   : Around joints, face and neck
May be deferred if necessary : Trunk, chest, abdomen, thighs

Preparation of Splints

Splints of Hexcelite or Aquaplast are prepared ready to be applied immediately at the end of the operation (see p.188).

Immediate Pre-operative Preparation

Careful thought about the conduct of the operation, before the patient is anaesthetized, and discussion with the members of the theatre team, will save valuable time while the patient is anaesthetized.

In particular, it is necessary to plan:
1 The order in which the procedures will follow each other,
2 The sites which are to be used as donor skin, and
3 The sites from which eschar will be removed.

Each team member should be fully occupied in useful tasks throughout the operation. When the skin is to be meshed or used as postage stamps, one member will be identified to do this, and may not be available to assist at the operation table itself.

Two instrument trollies are set, one for taking the skin graft, the other for carrying out the escharectomy. A third is required for dressings (Appendix, p.248).

Adequate quantities of vaseline tulle gras, dressings, wool and bandages are unwrapped ready on the nurses' trolley before the operation begins.

Four skin graft knives, two for desloughing and two for taking the donor autografts are set to an appropriate thickness of cut. Extra disposable blades are unwrapped ready for use. Time spent in waiting for appropriate instruments, dressings and suture materials to be brought from the clean utility room to the theatre means a lengthened time for anaesthesia.

In planning the operation, it is borne in mind that, in most cases, it is desirable to limit the blood loss to less than 30% of the circulating blood volume, and also, because of the poor anaesthetic risk these patients present, the operating time to less than 1 hour. This usually confines the escharectomy to a maximum of 30% body surface area. This implies that two, or, for a large burn, three nurses will need to be scrubbed, with at least two 'runners'. Sufficient surgeons need to be involved to reduce operating time to acceptable levels, but not so many as to impede each others' activities around the table. For a large burn, two surgeons, each with an assistant, are usually enough; a third is occupied preparing the grafts by mesher or cutting into postage stamps.

The surgeon who will apply the skin preparation antiseptic dons two pairs of gloves.

The Operation

In the heated operating room on the operating table, the dressings of the anaesthetized patient are entirely removed by 'runners' wearing sterile gloves. He is then laid naked on a large sterile towel.

Bacteriology swabs are taken from several sites by a 'runner'.

The electrodiathermy plate is applied.

The burned areas are cleaned by the surgeon with cetrimide 1% and chlorhexidine 0.05%, and covered with operating towels.

The surgeon removes the outer pair of gloves.

Using fresh uncontaminated antiseptic solutions, the donor skin graft areas are cleaned and left exposed.

Donor autografts, sufficient to cover the areas already planned for escharectomy, are removed with a skin graft knife (Fig. 14.1). The grafts are handed to a scrubbed surgeon away from the table. He meshes, spreads onto tulle gras or cuts them into postage stamps (Fig. 14.2). The donor wounds are dressed with vaseline tulle, gauze dressings, wool and bandaged, or with Opsite.

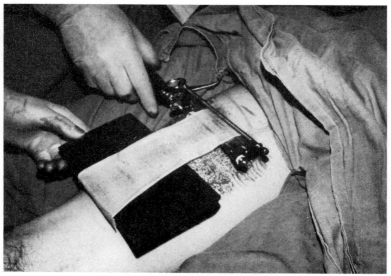

Fig. 14.1   Cutting a split skin graft

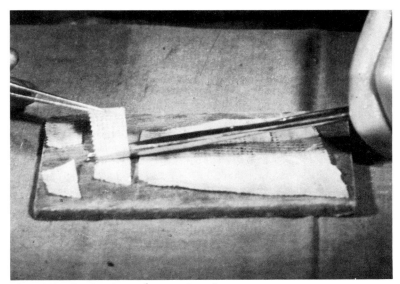

Fig. 14.2 Cutting 'postage stamp' grafts

The towels over the burned areas are removed, and eschar excised from such areas as have been previously planned. Scissors, forceps and a skin graft knife are employed for this purpose.

Techniques of Escharectomy

1 Excision using a skin grafting knife, set to about 0.025 cm (0.01 inch), the eschar is shaved off plane by plane. As soon as punctate bleeding is reached, the bed is sufficient to support an immediately applied graft. If allowed to dry out, this initially bleeding layer dies.

   This method of 'tangential shaving' is useful for areas such as the dorsum of the hand and fingers. It is satisfactorily combined with technique 2 for most other areas.

2 Sharp and blunt dissection. Using McIndoe or Mayo scissors, eschar is excised along a plane developed beneath the eschar initially by the blunt tip of the scissors. The excision is continued by a combination of blunt and sharp dissection, coagulating vessels as they bleed.

3 Avulsion of eschar. Eschar is secured in artery forceps or tissue-holding forceps. By applying traction, it is avulsed from the bed along a plane which leaves vessels which require coagulation. Haemostasis is secured. This somewhat 'indelicate' method is

favoured by some surgeons for burns of the thigh and abdomen.

Graft Application

The grafts are then applied and carefully secured either with sutures or a large sheet of vaseline tulle gras, not more than one layer thick. If near a joint, appropriate splintage is applied to immobilize the joint. Several thick layers of cotton wool may be sufficient, but for the legs or elbows, plaster of Paris or Hexcelite is more secure. To immobilize the shoulder, several layers of cotton wool and a spica bandage or a pre-formed Hexcelite splint are appropriate.

Those burned areas which have not been grafted are now cleaned with cetrimide – chlorhexidine, and redressed with Bactigras tulle or silver sulphadiazine.

The anaesthetic is ended.

Finally, on a drawing of a mannikin in the patient's notes, an accurate record is made of:

1 Which areas have been grafted;
2 Which areas have been desloughed but not grafted (if any);
3 The donor skin graft sites.

Graft Storage

Any unused autograft is laid under sterile conditions onto a layer of gauze which has been rung out in normal saline. The gauze containing the graft is rolled into a cigar shape, and stored in universal containers in the refrigerator at 4°C. The patient's name, and the date of operation are recorded on the container.

When several pieces of skin are to be stored, each should be placed into an individual container, so that when the skin is to be applied to the patient later in the ward, only those amounts of skin which are to be used will be removed from the refrigerator. Removal of skin from the refrigerator and then re-cooling is detrimental, and reduces the survival time of the stored skin.

Types of Graft

Full or Thick Partial-thickness Grafts

Eyelids almost always require thick partial-thickness or full-thickness grafts. The groove behind the ears between the pinna and the scalp is a useful source of full-thickness skin.

Full-thickness grafts are held in place on the eyelid by sutures, one end of which is left long. The graft is covered by a layer of tulle gras and a bolus of proflavine wool. The long suture ends are tied over the bolus to each other. (See p.181).

Fingers, especially on the flexor surfaces, also require full-thickness or thick partial-thickness grafts, to prevent flexion contracture; the thinner the graft the more it subsequently contracts. Elsewhere, almost without exception, partial thickness autografts are used.

Sheet Grafts

Small areas of burn, say up to 10×10 cm, may be covered by a continuous sheet of autograft, usually spread onto tulle gras for ease of application. It is useful to puncture such a sheet of graft with the point of scissors every 2 cm or so, to permit egress of serum or blood from beneath it. If the grafted wound can be protected from rubbing on the bed-clothes, it may be left exposed. Otherwise it will be dressed with tulle gras, gauze and bandages to prevent it shearing on the wound. When larger areas are to be grafted, the choice lies between meshed skin or 'postage stamps'.

Mesh Grafts

Sheets of autograft are cut into mesh on a 'Dermacarrier' or 'Meshgraft' dermatome to produce a chicken-wire appearance (Figs. 14.3 & 14.4). Expansion of the skin may be three or five times the original area, depending on the template used for meshing. The meshed graft is spread onto the wound, taking care that the epidermal side is uppermost. Epithelialization of the burned surface occurs from the margins of the mesh strips and by wound contracture. This latter makes the method unsatisfactory for use over joints.

The long-term appearance of the graft is more or less reticulated (Fig. 14.5) and is often cosmetically odd-looking. Mesh grafts are therefore best avoided for the face, hands and females' calves. Wear-and-tear characteristics of meshed autografts and their ability to withstand friction may be disappointing. They are, however, satisfactory for the chest, abdomen, back and upper thighs.

For extensive burns, meshing of grafts permits small areas of surviving donor skin to be used to cover quite large areas of burn.

If this method is used, it is always necessary to dress the grafted area with tulle gras or Bactigras tulle, or with homograft, in order to prevent the interstices between the mesh desiccating.

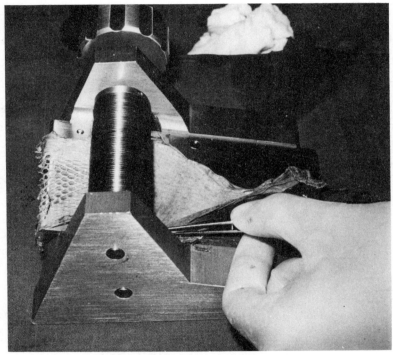

Fig. 14.3   The Skin Mesher

Postage-stamps

Donor autograft skin is laid onto tulle gras and together cut into squares or rectangles about 3 cm × 3 cm. The skin and tulle gras squares are laid onto the wound. Small gaps (0.5 – 1 cm) between the grafts are permissible. Thus burned areas larger than the area of donor skin can be grafted.

Serum or blood exudate escape around the margins of each stamp.

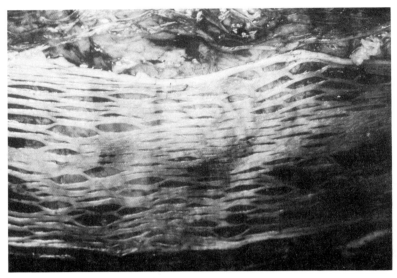

Fig. 14.4   Meshed skin graft

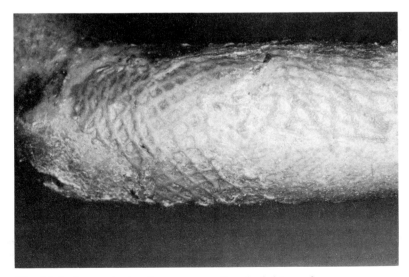

Fig. 14.5   Late reticulated appearance of meshed skin graft

Depending on the thickness of the grafts and the width of the intervening gaps between them contracture is much less than with mesh, and the wear-and-tear qualities are almost as good as sheet grafts.

Shearing of the grafts on the wound bed must be prevented by covering the whole grafted area with a single layer of tulle gras, and adequate immobilization, either by bandaging or splinting.

References

ARTZ, C.P., MONCRIEF, J.A. & PRUITT, B.A.(1979) *Burns – a Team Approach.* W.B. Saunders, Philadelphia.

BAXTER, C.R. & BURKE, J.(1984) Excision Therapy in Burn Injury. *J. Burn Care Rehab*, **5**, 430.

BERRY, R.B. & HACKETT, M.E.J.(1980) Evaluation of Lyophilized Homograft, Pigskin and Frozen Pigskin Biological Dressings. *Burns*, **7**, 84.

BURKE, J.F., BONDOC, C.C. & QUINBY, W.C.(1974) Primary Burn Excision and Immediate Grafting, *J. Trauma*, **14**, 389.

DOSSING, M. & SORENSEN, B.(1975) Freeze Dried and Non-freeze Dried Allografts on Excised Burns. *Burns*, **2**, 36.

EVANS, A.J.(1974) Surgical Aspects of Burns. *Proc. R. Soc. Med.*, **67**, 253.

GRANT, C.G., WARREN, R. & SALTER, E.(1980) Expansion of Skin *in vitro* for Grafting on to Extensive Burns. *Burns*, **7**, 57.

JANZEKOVIC, Z.(1977) Excisions of Burns. *Burns*, **4**, 61.

JURKIEWICZ, M.J.(1979) Excisional Therapy. *J. Trauma*, **19**, Suppl. 11, 933.

KEMBLE, J.V.H. & LAMB, B.E.(1984) *Plastic Surgical and Burns Nursing.* Baillière Tindall, London.

MACMILLAN, B.(1979) Depth of Injury. *J. Trauma*, **19**, Suppl. 11, 927.

MCDOUGALL, W.S., SLADE, C.L. & PRUITT, B.A.(1978) *Manual of Burns.* Springer, New York.

MOSEROVA, J. & HOUSKOVA, E.(1982) Histology of Early Necrectomy. *Burns*, **8**, 399.

SMAHEL, J. & CLODIUS L.(1983) Skin Wounds Covered with Mesh Graft. *Chir. Plast.*, **7**, 175.

SORENSEN, B.(1981) Acute Excision or Exposure Treatment? *Acta Chir. Plast. (Prague)*, **23**, 67.

STONE, H.H. & HOBBY, L.W.(1965) Use of the Mesh Dermatome for Major Burns. *American Surgeon (Philadelphia)*, **31**, 583.

TANDON, S.N. & SUTHERLAND, A.B.(1977) Problems following Tangential Excision and Skin Grafting in Dermal Burns. *Burns*, **3**, 96.

TANNER, J.C., VANDEPUT, J. & OLLEY, J.F.(1964) The Mesh Skin Graft. *Plast. Reconstruct. Surg.*, **34**, 287.

VISTNES, L.M.(1979) Methods of Excision. *J. Trauma*, **19**, Suppl. 11, 924.

WHITTAKER, A.H.(1953) Treatment of Burns by Excision and Immediate Grafting. *Am. J. Surg.*, **84**, 411.

15

Anaesthesia for the Burned Patient

General Anaesthesia for Excision and Grafting Procedures in Extensive Burns

This is a major surgical procedure and an adequate number of trained staff should be available to enable the operation to proceed expeditiously. Two anaesthetists are needed, as fluid replacement is a full-time activity for one person. It is important to limit the operating time to approximately one hour as this keeps the blood loss within manageable volumes, although twice the blood volume may be lost in this time. Also heat and energy loss from the exposure of the raw areas are thereby limited, especially if the theatre ambient temperature is raised.

There are several special problems associated with anaesthesia for a major excision and grafting procedure.

Timing of Operation and Premedication

This depends on the surgical decision regarding early or late excision. Tangential excision is usually carried out up to the 5th day. At the preoperative visit, the anaesthetist attempts to inspire confidence and trust in the patient and make an assessment of his general condition. The resuscitation phase should be complete and the patient should be haemodynamically stable and with good renal function. Inadequate gaseous exchange in a patient with respiratory burns or an intercurrent chest infection is a reason for postponement of operation to allow improvement in the chest condition. Systemic infection and a raised temperature are not contraindications, as removal of the dead tissue may improve this situation.

Adequate supplies of blood must be available. Eight units should be ordered intially for a major burn exceeding 15% body surface area and the laboratory should be forewarned that more may be required. There is little advantage in attempting to raise the haemoglobin preoperatively but additional blood will be needed if this is already low. The routine use of platelet and fresh frozen plasma infusions to prevent clotting problems precludes the need for fresh blood. If plasma reduced blood is provided, additional crystalloid solutions should be given to make up the volume deficit.

The feeding regime of the patient is interrupted for the minimal period preoperatively (4 hours, irrespective of the presence of a Ryle's tube) and adequate premedication with papaveretum and hyoscine is given one hour before the anticipated theatre time, as movement from bed to operating table may be very painful.

Induction and Establishment of the Airway

Anaesthesia is induced with intravenous thiopentone if the face and neck have not been injured, followed by intubation using non-depolarizing muscle relaxants. However, if the face is burned it may become extremely awkward to maintain an air-tight fit with a mask, even padded with wet gauze swabs and the airway may be lost. The mandible may be fixed by eschar at an early stage although eschar can be broken in order to mobilise the tongue and clear the airway. Burned skin is slippery, greasy and unaesthetic and it can be difficult to hold the laryngoscope or squeeze the rebreathing bag after holding the mask on the face.

In this situation, one anaesthetist is concerned with the airway and preoxygenating the patient, while a second person inserts a small indwelling needle. Inhalational anaesthesia proceeds using nitrous oxide, oxygen and enflurane, and when anaesthesia is deep enough, the mouth and pharynx are inspected. It is shown that it is possible to inflate the chest using a mask before any muscle relaxant drugs are given. Most major burn procedures require intubation and ventilation. The advantages are that the airway is established; it allows for change of position to reach burns on the back; and it reduces the oxygen requirements associated with deep rapid spontaneous respiration in a patient in a highly catabolic state after a burn.

Drugs

Depolarizing muscle relaxants

Suxamethonium is not often used in burned patients. Reports of cardiac arrest following administration of suxamethonium are associated with a rise in serum potassium and are maximal around the 49th day post-burn. This may not be the only factor involved, as there are low serum cholinesterase levels and changes at the muscle end plate that affect the pharmacology after burn injury. (Suxamethonium may be used for intubation in the immediate post-burn period.)

Non-depolarizing muscle relaxants

There is an increased dose requirement for these drugs. Pancuronium (dose 6–8 mg for intubation and increments of 2 mg as required IV) or atracurium (dose 0.6 mg/kg for intubation and increments of 0.3 mg/kg IV) are the drugs of choice. (Tubocurarine may be associated with a fall in blood pressure due to histamine release.) The shorter action of pancuronium and atracurium is due to increased plasma binding and to changes at the neuromuscular junction. There is usually no difficulty in reversing muscular relaxation in those patients using neostigmine 2.5 mg with atropine 1.2 mg.

Analgesics

Pain is a major feature especially postoperatively. Donor areas are always painful and grafted areas are painful if moved. Intraoperatively, phenoperidine 1–2 mg IV repeated after 45 minutes, or fentanyl 0.05 – 0.1 mg IV repeated after 30 minutes are given.

Hypnotics

Hypnosis is achieved using nitrous oxide, which is also a mild analgesic, and an inhalational agent such as enflurane or halothane. As repeated anaesthetics are common, enflurane is the drug of choice at present.

Opportunities to Minimize Bleeding

Excessive bleeding is of such importance during burns surgery that methods of reducing blood loss are sought. Excision of limb burns can sometimes be performed under tourniquet or with the limb elevated. Hypotensive anaesthesia has been used but it is impracticable due to the difficulties with monitoring.

Fluid Replacement

Lack of veins can be a serious problem in a large burn and a good IV line is of pre-eminent importance. A large cannula (14 gauge) should be inserted, preferably through unburned skin and a free-running drip established with clear fluid. The tubing should run through a blood warmer and a pressure bag should be available to speed the flow. A second drip may be required and if necessary a cut-down should be done at this stage.

Excision of 1% of the body surface can lose 100 mls of blood or more and so the treatment of 15 – 20% of burned skin in one session lasting one hour will require the replacement of about 2.5 litres of blood. This is nearly the maximum that can be administered through one 14-gauge cannula in an hour. At the end of the operation, oozing occurs and the haemoglobin continues to fall, so 2 – 3 extra units should be given slowly in the postoperative period. Consequently, these patients receive massive blood transfusions.

Complications of Massive Blood Transfusion

Temperature

Cold blood transfusion causes hypothermia and may cause cardiac arrest. The infused blood is heated to 36°C by an in-line warming device (water bath or dry heat warmer).

Calcium, citrate and potassium

In stored blood there are high concentrations of potassium ions and citrate but no free calcium ions. Calcium counteracts the toxic effects of citrate and is the physiological antagonist of potassium. Calcium chloride or gluconate 1 g IV should be given if the infusion rate is very rapid especially as calcium metabolism is altered in the post-burn state. A fall in blood pressure unresponsive to increased volume administraton may respond to an injection of calcium gluconate.

Acid-base changes

Although stored blood is acidic, there is no indication for the administration of sodium bicarbonate because citrate metabolism generates bicarbonate. A progressive metabolic alkalosis occurs.

Abnormalities of clotting

After a transfusion equivalent to the initial blood volume, only 25% of the original blood will be circulating. Old stored blood has no viable platelets and little Factor V and VIII activity. Decaying platelets and old red and white cells form microaggregates which act as thromboplastins and destroy clotting factors. Diffuse intravascular coagulation (DIC) and failure of coagulation becomes more likely with large volume transfusions. Filtration of blood with filters of pore size 20 – 40 μm removes the larger microaggregates. However, the use of these filters tends to slow the rate of infusion, even when a pressure bag is used. The filter requires changing after 2 – 3 units and the use of two giving sets and a 3-way tap can help to speed up the changeover.

After half the blood volume has been replaced, six units of concentrated platelets and 1 unit of fresh frozen plasma, (FFP) which will provide the labile clotting factors, should be given. This prevents the development of abnormal clotting. (See p.80).

Monitoring

This is often minimal due to lack of access. Limbs may be burned or if not, may be required as donor sites. There may be a lack of large superficial veins, and intra-arterial lines are undesirable because of the infection risk. In practice:

1 *ECG* Leads should be applied where possible. If necessary, needle electrodes can be used through burned tissue.
2 *Blood pressure* If possible a cuff is applied to an unburned limb. If the area is needed as a donor site, the cuff can be applied over the bandage after harvesting the skin.
3 *Temperature* Comparison of temperature readings from a skin probe (shell) and pharyngeal probe (core) help to indicate the adequacy of transfusion.
4 *CVP* If a vein is available for central venous cannulation, this measurement is useful in ascertaining the adequacy of transfusion.
5 *Blood loss* A visual assessment is made of the volume of blood on the swabs allowing for the use of saline. Weighing of swabs is rather inaccurate under these conditions.

Post-operative Care

Good analgesia, preferably given intravenously, is essential and a fluid and blood regime is ordered to provide an adequate postoperative haemoglobin. Normal eating and drinking should be encouraged as soon as possible.

General Anaesthesia for Excision of Burns in Children

All the factors that apply to general anaesthesia in an adult burned patient need consideration in children. Because of the size of the child certain factors become more important.

Venous Access

All children having a grafting procedure, however small, should have an IV line. Apart from replacement of blood lost in surgery, they need IV fluid because of preoperative fasting. Postoperatively, they often do not drink well and urine output may fall. It also provides an opportunity to top-up haemoglobin to aid healing.

Scalp vein cannulation is not suitable for blood replacement at the rate required during surgery. A cut-down is done if no suitable superficial vein can be found.

Replacement of Blood Loss

Accurate volume replacement is very important in a small child. Figure 15.1 shows a simple system of blood administration in a baby. Alternatively a volumetric pump may be used.

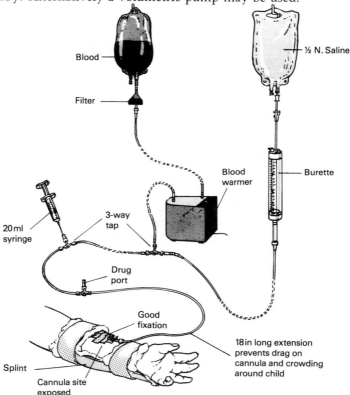

Fig. 15.1　Apparatus for administration of precise volumes of warm, filtered blood to babies

The blood volume is calculated:

Blood volume in ml = 80 × weight in kg.
($\frac{1}{10}$ blood volume is equivalent to 0.5 l in an adult)

Blood is replaced when one-tenth blood volume is lost. If the child is anaemic preoperatively, a one-tenth blood volume transfusion raises the haemoglobin by 1 g. Blood should be replaced as it is lost and the surgeon must stop excision and apply pressure, until the estimated loss is transfused. Careful note is kept of the volume given. Blood replacement should be done in theatre where it is the anaesthetist's responsibility. Blood to raise haemoglobin can continue in the ward. It is easier to calculate the volume requirements, if whole blood is used and fresh blood prevents coagulation problems in what may be virtually an exchange transfusion.

Heat Loss

The surface area relative to mass of a child is greater than of an adult. Heat losses are therefore relatively greater and temperature regulation may be disturbed in a small sick baby. The child lies on a heating blanket and any unburned parts, or those not needed as donor areas including the scalp, are wrapped in aluminium foil.

Ventilation

The child should be intubated after atropine premedication and intermittent positive pressure ventilation (IPPV) carried out by hand using a modified T piece or a suitable ventilator, e.g. Penlon with Newton valve. One anaesthetist should be responsible for the airway and ventilation and one for fluid replacement.

Drugs

Suxamethonium should not be used. Pancuronium is used for relaxation, dose 0.1 mg/kg (supplementary doses ¼ the initial dose) or atracurium (dose 0.5 mg/kg). Fentanyl is used for analgesia, dose 1 μg/kg. Relation is reversed with neostigmine 0.05 mg/kg and atropine 0.02 mg/kg.

Monitoring

Temperature, blood pressure and ECG are monitored and the use of a praecordial stethoscope is advised.

Anaesthesia for Dressings and Minor Procedures

This may be a frequent occurrence and so the co-operation of the patient is essential. There should be minimal disruption of the feeding regime.

General Anaesthesia

Thiopentone induction and nitrous oxide, oxygen and enflurane are administered via a mask and spontaneous respiration.

Self-administered Inhalational Analgesia

e.g. Entonox (50% N_2O/O_2) or
Low concentrations of enflurane in air using a draw-over vaporizer.
Higher concentrations of nitrous oxide may be administered by an anaesthetist using a Quantiflex apparatus or an anaesthetic machine.

Intravenous Analgesia

Ketamine

The patient is prepared as though for a general anaesthetic. Atropine is given before IV or IM ketamine. An anaesthetist should be present.
Dose: IM 5–10 mg/kg – lasts 15 min.
IV 1–4 mg/kg – lasts 5–10 min.
Supplementary dose 0.5 mg/kg.

Special Conditions Requiring Early Operation and Anaesthesia

Escharotomy

Deep dermal or full-thickness burns

Relaxation incisions may be required in circumferential burns of limbs where the eschar is producing a tourniquet effect or if respiratory embarrassment results from extensive burns of chest and neck. Usually no anaesthetic is required as the tissue is dead and painless.

Electrical burns

General anaesthesia is required for relaxation incisions through relatively normal skin to open deep muscle compartments (fasciotomy). The electrical current passes along the fascial planes and along nerves and blood vessels which have low resistance, and destruction and muscle necrosis often extends much further than at first appears. The passage of current through the body may have passed through and damaged the heart. Irritability of the myocardium with raised cardiac enzymes, and ECG changes may follow. Myocardial infarction has been reported during recovery from an electrical burn.

Operations on Special Functional Areas

Very early operation may be indicated to preserve function, e.g. eyelids and hands. Particular attention must be paid to maintaining blood pressure during anaesthesia in the resuscitation phase.

General Anaesthesia for Intubation or Tracheostomy

This may be required in a patient with respiratory obstruction (see Chapter 16).

Pain Relief

Early sedation and analgesia given intravenously help to allay the fear and pain associated with extensive burns. Patients with full-thickness burns may not complain of severe pain because the sensory nerve endings in the skin have been destroyed. Restlessness and confusion due to hypoxaemia or hypovolaemia should be distinguished from pain and treated accordingly.

Drugs

1 IV Morphine. Does $0.1 - 0.2$ mg/kg given as a diluted solution 10 mg in 10 mls of water by a doctor and titrated against the patient's conditon.
2 IV Chlorpromazine. Dose 0.5 mg/kg diluted to 50 mg/10 ml. Repeated 6 hourly. This potentiates the effect of morphine and is antiemetic and sedative. It is best avoided in children because of its rare association with the neuroleptic malignant syndrome.

General Anaesthesia for Late Complications of Burns

Contractures of skin and hypertrophic scarring may require release months or years after the initial injury. Z-plasty may be used to lengthen the scars or full thickness skin grafts applied. More extensive reconstruction with flaps may be needed. The patients who present special difficulty to the anaesthetist are those with severe contractures of the neck and face or with microstoma. Incision of the contractures is required before intubation can be carried out.

Method. Ketamine anaesthesia is used until sufficient mobility is provided by incision of the contractures to allow endotracheal intubation. After analgesic and atropine premedication, IV ketamine 2 mg/kg is given. Anaesthesia occurs in 30 seconds and lasts for 5 – 10 minutes. Supplementary doses of 0.5 mg/kg are given until conditions are suitable for intubation, after preoxygenation and IV suxamethonium provided at least 3 months have passed since the burn injury. Anaesthesia can then continue in the normal way. It should be remembered that ketamine anaesthesia does not guarantee protection of the airway against aspiration but respiration is not depressed except by large doses.

References

BROWN, J.M. (1985) Aspects of Thermal Injury. *Recent Adv. Anaesth. Analg.,* **15**, 155.

BUSH, G.H., GRAHAM, H.A.P., LITTLEWOOD, A.H.M. & SCOTT, L.B.(1962) Danger of Suxamethonium and Endotracheal Intubation in Anaesthesia for Burns. *Bri. Med. J.,* **ii**, 1081.

DIAMOND, A.W., PIGGOT, R.W. & TOWNSEND, P.L.G.(1975) Immediate Care of Burns. *Anaesthesia,* **30**, 791.

FILKINS, S.A., COSGRAVE, P. *et al* (1981) Self-administered Anaesthetic for Pain Control *J. Burn Care Rehab.,* **2**, 33.

FIRN, S. (1982) Enflurane Analgesia. *J. R. Soc. Med., Suppl.,* 1, **75**, 36.

HORSEY, P.J. (1982) Blood transfusion. *Recent Adv. Anaesth. Analg.,* **14**, 89.

POOLE-WILSON, P.A. (1978) Clinical Interpretation of Haemodynamic Measurements. *Br. J. Hosp. Med.,* **204**, 371.

WILLIAMS, J.G., RILEY, T.R.D. & MOODY, R.A. (1983) Resuscitation Experience in the Falkland Islands Campaign. *Br. Med. J.,* **286**, 775.

16

Intensive Care of the Patient with Respiratory Burns

The anaesthetist is involved when respiratory function is diminished by inhalational injury. The presence of respiratory damage in a patient with a burn is the most important single factor affecting mortality.

Any degree of inhalational damage may cause hypoxaemia and this is aggravated by hypovolaemia and hypotension which may occur during the resuscitation phase. Red cell destruction in burned skin reduces oxygen carriage by haemoglobin compounding the problem; there is an increased oxygen requirement at cellular level during the catabolic phase.

Mechanisms of Hypoxaemia Associated with Inhalational Damage

Direct Thermal or Chemical Injury to the Respiratory Tract

External

Tissue oedema following burns of the face, neck and trunk interferes with respiration. Swelling of the face and neck leads to direct obstruction of the upper airway. Swelling of the tongue and fixation of the mandible cause pharyngeal obstruction. These patients need urgent intubation or if this is not possible, tracheostomy. Early mild airway obstruction usually worsens and therefore intubation should be considered before a crisis develops.

Escharotomy is required for circumferential burns of the trunk which prevent free respiratory movements, and for burns of the neck where enclosed oedema may cause tracheal obstruction.

Upper respiratory tract

Hot dry air cools rapidly and thus the internal damage from this is usually confined to the respiratory tract above the vocal cords. Mucosal oedema results in narrowing of the airway; more severe damage results in exudation and ulceration.

Lower respiratory tract

This is more frequently affected by steam or explosion releasing hot or toxic gas. Since water has a high heat carrying capacity, it may still be hot when it reaches the alveoli. This causes an inflammatory exudate with interstitial and alveolar oedema, and thickening of the alveolar walls reducing gaseous exchange. Thermal injury may lead to ciliary damage or a deficiency of surfactant. This substance lowers the surface tension of the walls of the alveoli which helps to maintain their patency. A deficiency of surfactant leads to collapse of alveoli.

An explosion in a confined space may cause pressure effects on the lung tissue. Pneumothorax, pulmonary oedema from alveolar damage and surgical emphysema of the mediastinum may occur. Septicaemia is an early complication, possibly due to the formation of alveolar–venous fistulae with direct access to the blood stream for infected material.

Carbon Monoxide Poisoning

Carbon monoxide is produced by the incomplete combustion of carbon, and occurs when a fire has developed in a confined space. Carbon monoxide has no taste or smell, and when inhaled, combines with haemoglobin to form carboxyhaemoglobin. Carbon monoxide has an affinity for haemoglobin which is 200 times that of oxygen and so displaces oxygen carried in the blood by haemoglobin. This leads to tissue hypoxia. Classically, patients with carbon monoxide poisoning are cherry pink in colour, although they are anoxic. Carboxyhaemoglobin levels of 5% are commonly found in burned patients on admission. Unconsciousness develops at a carboxy-haemoglobin level of 30%. In these patients the bronchial tree may be normal. The treatment is with oxygen, if necessary by intermittent positive pressure ventilation.

Smoke Inhalation Including Toxic Fumes

Hypoxia may occur due to depletion of the available oxygen in the air when combustion takes place in a confined space or when the inhalation of smoke displaces oxygen from the inspired air. Inhaled smoke or chemical irritants may produce severe pulmonary oedema and bronchospasm or may interfere with capillary permeability. The direct toxic effects of gases produced when modern materials ignite, may also be lethal. Polyurethane foam, widely used as a filler in modern furniture, gives off smoke containing isocyanates which break down to hydrogen cyanate, carbon monoxide and ammonia. At 1000°C, hydrogen cyanide is produced. Death from cyanide poisoning occurs at a serum level of about 100 μmol/l. Cyanide is a cellular poison.

The types of anoxia are summarized in Table 16.1.

Recognition and Diagnosis of the Extent of the Injury

History

A description of the scene of the fire should be obtained from eyewitnesses or the attending ambulancemen. The presence of smoke, steam, toxic fumes, flames near the face, whether there was an explosion or whether the fire was in a confined space help one to assess the problem presented by the patient.

Examination

Noisy respiration is highly significant and always indicates some element of obstruction to the airway. Stridor or wheezing on inspiration suggest upper airway obstruction, and expiratory wheezing lower airway involvement.

Early examination may show none of these signs but burns of the face, neck or mouth, singed hairs in the nose, and soot in the throat and nasopharynx are highly suggestive of respiratory injury. Such patients should be carefully observed for the development of obvious respiratory signs and symptoms which may take several hours to appear. Anticipation of oedema and intubation before it occurs may be life saving.

Investigations at this time often prove nothing. Chest X-ray and arterial gases may be normal and require to be repeated. Fibre-optic bronchoscopy is the most helpful additional investigation. The presence of soot and reddening within the bronchial tree confirms respiratory involvement.

Table 16.1 Summary of types of anoxia

Table	Example	Cyanosis	Blood gases
Anoxic	a) Low inspired oxygen e.g. Smoke inhalation Depletion by combustion of available O_2	Central	$PaO_2 \downarrow$
	b) Reduction in alveolar ventilation e.g. Respiratory obstruction – circumferential burns of trunk	Central	$PaO_2 \downarrow$ $PaCO_2 \uparrow$
	c) Impaired diffusion and distribution due to imbalance of blood supply and effective alveoli e.g. Pulmonary oedema (from thermal damage or smoke), Infection	Central	$PaO_2 \downarrow$
	d) Venous–Arterial shunts e.g. Pulmonary oedema, infection	Central	$PaO_2 \downarrow$
Anaemic	a) Low haemoglobin e.g. Pre-existing state. Destruction of red cells After skin grafting procedures During healing	No cyanosis	PaO_2 normal. (Total O_2 in blood $\downarrow$ PaO_2 depends on O_2 in solution)
	b) CO poisoning. CO displaces O_2 in Hb	Cherry pink	PaO_2 normal
Stagnant	Due to inadequate blood flow through tissues. e.g. Shock Hypovolaemia	Peripheral cyanosis	PaO_2 normal (Mixed venous $pO_2 \downarrow$ $\therefore$ excessive extraction of O_2 in tissues)
Histotoxic	Due to poisoning of intracellular enzymes. e.g. Cyanide poisoning from inhaling fumes from foam furniture Septicaemic shock	No cyanosis	PaO_2 normal Mixed venous $PO_2 \uparrow \therefore$ failure to extract O_2 in tissues

Management

The aim is to maintain respiratory exchange until healing has taken place in the lungs and to prevent the development of complications such as infection.

Observation

Admission to hospital is advisable for all patients who have inhaled smoke or have a history suggestive of a respiratory burn. Temperature, pulse and respiration rate is monitored 4 hourly. The chest is examined for the subsequent development of respiratory obstruction, pulmonary oedema or diffuse airways obstruction. Chest X-ray is done on admission and repeated after 24 hours. Sputum is examined for carbon deposits. Serial blood gas measurements may be helpful. Clinical evidence of central cyanosis and signs of cerebral hypoxia indicate a severe deterioration. The brain is particularly susceptible to oxygen lack and symptoms such as restlessness, disorientation and confusion may develop. Sequential peak flow estimations help to differentiate hypoxaemia due to diffuse airways obstruction from alveolar lesions.

Oxygen Therapy

The aim of oxygen therapy is to deliver more oxygen to tissues in a state of hypoxia.

Indications for oxygen therapy

1 Central cyanosis due to obstruction or inhalational damage.
2 Peripheral cyanosis due to hypotension and hypovolaemia.
3 Signs of cerebral hypoxia.
4 PaO_2 less than 10.6 kPa.
5 Carbon monoxide poisoning.

Method of administration of oxygen with spontaneous respiration

High concentrations of O_2
The MC (Mary Catterall) mask is a disposable face mask which is used to deliver concentrations of between 40 and 80%. A flow of 6 l/min gives 60% O_2.
Controlled concentrations of O_2
The ventimask, which works on the venturi principle with oxygen entrained in air, is a useful method of giving controlled concen-

trations of oxygen. Concentrations of 40%, 35%, 28% and 24% are possible and the concentration is adjusted by means of a colour-coded attachment. This is particularly useful during the recovery phase when the inspired oxygen concentration may gradually be reduced to that of air.

Humidification

Normally the nose acts as a humidifier, warming, filtering and humidifying inspired air. In a patient with a respiratory burn, the nasal mucosa may be damaged and unable to perform this function. After endotracheal intubation or tracheostomy where the nose is bypassed, humidification of inspired gases is mandatory. Dehydration of the airways leads to a reduction in ciliary activity and defective clearing of the tenacious secretions, and is made worse by systemic dehydration. At worst, this may lead to obstruction of a tracheostomy or endotracheal tube.

Various types of humidifier are used:
1 Water humidifiers, where gases are blown over the surface of warm water;
2 Gas driven nebulizers which produce a super-saturated mist with droplets of 5–20 μm
3 Ultrasonic nebulizers which give even smaller-sized water particles. Nebulizers are useful for the administration of bronchodilator drugs (e.g. salbutamol) in patients with diffuse airways obstruction. Mucolytic drugs (e.g. Tyloxapol) may also be administered in this way.

Physiotherapy

Physiotherapy of the chest is designed to improve the pattern of breathing and to assist coughing which helps to clear the major bronchi of secretions. Planned posture changes are used to aid bronchial drainage, and bagging and suction are carried out two or three times per day in patients with an endotracheal or tracheostomy tube. This is a combination of chest physiotherapy, manual ventilation and endotracheal suction. If the aspirate is very thick, 5 ml of normal saline are instilled into the trachea and suction repeated.

Endotracheal intubation

Indications

1 Evidence of obstruction of the upper respiratory tract or anticipation that this might occur when oedema develops. Stridor,

paradoxical respiration and the use of accessory muscles of respiration are all signs of obstruction.

2 To facilitate the removal of secretions from the bronchial tree.

3 To enable mechanical ventilation to be used.

Method

General anaesthesia allows better conditions for assessment of the extent of the injury and adequate suction of the pharynx and bronchial tree. Induction of anaesthesia should be by inhalation as the airway must not be further jeopardized by using respiratory depressant drugs or muscle relaxants.

Reflex vagal activity is reduced with IV atropine 0.6 mg. After preoxygenation, progressing to halothane and oxygen anaesthesia, a laryngoscope is inserted and the condition of the mouth, pharynx and larynx are examined by direct vision. Topical analgesia is applied using a lignocaine spray. If it is possible to inflate the chest using a mask, suxamethonium 75 mg. IV may be given to relax the vocal cords and ease intubation. An oral plastic tube with high volume, low pressure cuff is inserted. It may be necessary to use a smaller tube than normal at this stage, due to oedema. The tube is carefully fixed in position with a bandage around the neck; adhesive tape rarely remains in place on burned skin. The cuff on the tube is inflated until the leak is abolished. The volume of air required is recorded. The tube is secured in the correct position ensuring good air entry to both lungs. Any excess length should be cut off, or it may accidentally slip back. The level of the tube end may be seen when a chest X-ray is next performed.

Once the airway is established, depending on the size of the endotracheal tube, a fibreoptic bronchoscope may be passed through the tube and the condition of the lower respiratory tract ascertained.

Management of the intubated patient

1 Good fixation of the tube in the correct position.

2 Humidification — necessary because the nose and mouth have been bypassed.

3 Bronchial suction — as required using a sterile technique.

4 Oxygen-enriched air.

5 Physiotherapy — to aid bronchial toilet.

6 Toleration of the tube. Sick patients tolerate tubes well, but if this is a problem, sedation is needed and respiratory depression may result, requiring intermittent positive pressure ventilation (IPPV).

7 Deflation of the cuff. By using low-pressure, high-volume cuffed tubes, there is less likelihood of damage to the laryngeal or tracheal mucosa. Therefore deflation is only necessary once in 24 hours, to

check that the same volume of air is required to ensure a seal. If a larger volume is needed it may mean that the oedema has subsided and either a larger tube can be inserted or even that extubation can be performed.

8 Changing of tube and extubation. A short general anaesthetic may be required, especially in children. After extubation, if respiration is quiet and there is no sign of obstruction, the tube need not be replaced.

9 Prolonged intubation. Endotracheal tubes have been left in position for up to 3 weeks without damage to the larynx. Tracheostomy is undesirable in burned patients because of the easier access to the bronchial tree it presents for infection, and it should be postponed as long as possible.

Tracheostomy

Tracheostomy allows better fixation of the tube, greater patient tolerance and easier bronchial toilet, but it provides more direct access for infection, especially if the neck is burned.

Indications

1 Obstruction of the airway due to burns of the face, tongue or pharynx in which it is impossible to insert an oral endotracheal tube.
2 After 3 weeks endotracheal intubation.
3 To allow supraglottal healing which has been prevented by the presence of an oral endotracheal tube.

Management of a patient with a tracheostomy

This is similar to the care of a patient with an endotracheal tube. The tracheostomy tube may need to be changed it if becomes blocked due to crusting of secretions. If the sputum is thick and infected, it needs changing every few days.

Intermittent Positive Pressure Ventilation

Control of respiration with intermittent positive pressure ventilation is required in patients with respiratory failure.

Indications for IPPV

1 Failure of adequate gaseous exchange as shown by:
   (a) hypoxaemia. PaO_2 less than $8\,kPa$ with inspired oxygen concentration of 50%.

(b) $PaCO_2$ above 7.5 kPa and rising.
(c) Falling pH.
(d) Increased respiratory rate.
(e) Increased pulse rate.
(f) Cyanosis.
(g) Irritability and restlessness.

2 Exhaustion of the patient and an inability to cough as a result of the increase in the effort of breathing.

3 The use of sedative drugs to enable toleration of an endotracheal tube, resulting in respiratory depression.

4 Pulmonary oedema (frothy blood-stained sputum) if uncontrolled by diuretic therapy.

Method

A ventilator with easily sterilizable patient circuit is prepared. A humidifier is connected and the required concentration of oxygen in air is set. In the average adult, the ventilator adjustments are fixed to give a respiratory rate of between 10 and 15 breaths/minute and the tidal volume between 600 and 800 ml. Allowance is made for weight and sex. The machine is switched on and tested for leaks.

After explaining what is happening to the patient, a muscle relaxant drug is given IV to stop the patient breathing and control of respiration is effected manually using a rebreathing bag. This allows the anaesthetist to assess the compliance of the chest and to determine the amount of pressure required to give adequate chest movement. The patient is then connected to the ventilator via the endotracheal or tracheostomy tube and a catheter mount. Movements of the chest are observed and air entry is confirmed by auscultation. The inflation pressure on the ventilator is noted and any adjustments of volume, rate and flow are made. Excessive inflation pressure may cause a fall in blood pressure and damage to the lungs including pneumothorax. Inflation pressure should rarely exceed 40 cm H_2O. A moderate amount of hyperventilation is often used which in itself helps to control respiration. A note is made of the ventilator settings and the patient reassessed after 15 minutes on the ventilator.

Drugs used in the control of ventilation

1 Muscle relaxants, e.g. pancuronium bromide. Route IV initial dose 6 mg. Increments of 2 mg as required about 1 hourly. These drugs are useful to control the situation initially but are undesirable for long term IPPV, as it is not pleasant for a patient to be conscious and unable to move.

2 Narcotic analgesics e.g. phenoperidine. Route IV. Dose 2–4 mg

given 2–4 hourly. This depresses respiration centrally and relieves pain, but patients can move and respond to instructions.

3 Sedatives and hypnotics e.g. diazepam 5–10 mg 6 hourly or chlorpromazine 0.5 mg/kg 6 hourly. Route IM or orally via nasogastric tube. These drugs alleviate fear and also potentiate the analgesic effect of narcotics and suppress nausea and vomiting.

Management of a Patient on a Ventilator

Care related to the patient's general condition

A patient being ventilated is not necessarily unconscious and all activities related to his case should be explained to him. Discussion of his condition should not continue as though he cannot hear. A patient on a ventilator should never be left unattended.

1 Normal hygiene.
2 Regular turning and positioning of patient and attention to pressure areas.
3 Urinary catheter.
4 Nasogastric tube for feeding.
5 Normal fluid balance and dietary requirements.
6 Physiotherapy to the chest and passive movements of all joints.
7 Monitoring of pulse, temperature, ECG and blood pressure. IPPV may cause a fall in BP especially if the patient is hypovolaemic.
8 IV lines. All patients being ventilated should have an IV line for administration of drugs and fluid requirements and to allow for immediate treatment of a fall in blood pressure.
9 Administration of drugs regularly and as required.
10 Chest X-ray, 3 times per week or more often if required.
11 Blood gases are measured daily or more frequently if the condition is unstable. The aim is to maintain PaO_2 between 10 and 12 kPa and $PaCO_2$ normal or slightly low i.e. 3–5.6 kPa. If the desired PaO_2 can only be maintained by ventilation producing a low $PaCO_2$, added dead space can be included in the circuit by lengthening the catheter mount. The minimum inspired oxygen concentrations to produce these levels should be used.

Care relating to the ventilator

1 Fixation of the endotracheal tube.
2 Support of the hoses of the ventilator so that they do not drag on the endotracheal tube.
3 Drainage of the condensate. Water vapour from the humidifier tends to condense on the inside of the tubes and this must be drained periodically.

4 Humidifer: The temperature and fluid level are checked regularly.
5 Equipment is available for manual ventilation in case of machine failure, gas leaks or accidental disconnection. Alternative endotracheal or tracheostomy tubes should be nearby in case of obstruction.
6 Monitoring of ventilator settings is performed hourly, i.e. rate, tidal volume, minute volume, inspiratory pressure, inspired oxygen concentration.
7 Continuous measurement of end tidal CO_2 is possible with a simple connection in the ventilator circuit. ET CO_2 is virtually equal to $PaCO_2$ and this information simplifies the adjustment of ventilation.

Positive End Expiratory Pressure (PEEP)

Indications for PEEP

If the PaO_2 remains low despite a high inspired oxygen concentration, PEEP is indicated. A PEEP valve can be attached to most ventilators. If PaO_2 is lower than 7 kPa on 50% inspired oxygen, 5–10 cm H_2O of PEEP is applied. Moderate PEEP may be less dangerous than raising the inspired oxygen concentration.

Contraindications to PEEP

Hypovolaemia is an absolute contraindication and leads to a fall in cardiac output. Patients with diffuse airways obstruction should probably not be given PEEP and in pulmonary oedema it may lead to increased fluid retention in the lung and exacerbate the condition. Additional monitoring is necessary. Chest measurements are repeated to check for progressive air trapping and CXR to detect pneumothorax. Regular PaO_2 and urine output measurements are made.

Weaning off the ventilator

It is nearly always easier to commence artificial ventilation than to stop it. Weaning should be attempted when the original disease process for which IPPV was instituted has healed. The patient should be able to cough; chest compliance, assessed by manual ventilation and inflation pressure measurements, should be normal, and infection should be cleared. The chest X-ray and PaO_2 on an inspired oxygen of 25% should be normal.

Method

All sedative drugs and muscle relaxants are stopped during the night. In the morning the ventilator is disconnected and the patient encouraged to breathe. Careful observation of the adequacy of ventilation and for signs of respiratory distress or exhaustion is made. If necessary, IPPV is recommenced. Increasingly prolonged periods off the ventilator are tried until eventually the patient can breathe spontaneously all the time.

Weaning may be a simple process or may take several days to achieve. Certain aspects of the burned patient make weaning more difficult. Systemic infection, weight loss due to the prolonged catabolic state and fatigue all tend to delay satisfactory weaning. Loss of body weight causes weakness of the respiratory muscles. Body weight loss of 30% causes a 40% loss of diaphragmatic mass. Consequently, the general physical state of the patient should be as good as possible before weaning is attempted.

Use of Other Drugs

Steroids

The general view is that one large dose of hydrocortisone (1500–3000 mg) on admission with respiratory burns is helpful. Long-term steroid therapy interferes with healing and facilitates infection.

Antibiotics

Prophylactic antibiotic therapy is not used. Specific treatment is indicated if a pulmonary infection develops.

Bronchodilators

If diffuse airways obstruction is a feature of the respiratory condition, bronchodilator drugs are indicated. Salbutamol is given by nebulizer and aminophylline by IV infusion or as a bolus injection. The management of a patient with respiratory burn injury is summarized in Table 16.2.

Additional respiratory complications in patients with burn injury

Respiratory Infection

Infection from the burned skin or other organisms may cause

Table 16.2 Summary of management of patient with respiratory burn injury

Signs and symptoms	Action	Investigation
Noisy respiration History of inhalation damage	OBSERVATION $\longrightarrow \downarrow$ SPONTANEOUS RESPIRATION 35% O_2 by VENTIMASK HUMIDIFICATION $\downarrow$	
Serious suspicion of obstruction before swelling occurs	INCREASE O_2 to 50% (MC mask) (Bronchodilators) $\longleftarrow$ $\downarrow$	Falling PaO_2 <10 kPa
Swelling of face	GA (Inhalational) $\longleftarrow$ Full visual assessment $\downarrow$	PaO_2<8 kPa
Dyspnoea Stridor Fixed mandible	INTUBATION (Emergency surgery) $\downarrow$	
Restlessness Pain Inc. work of breathing ∴ Inc. O_2 requirements	ANALGESIA SEDATION RELAXATION $\longleftarrow$ IPPV	PaO_2<7 kPa $PaCO_2 \uparrow$
	PEEP 5 cm H_2O $\longleftarrow$ $\downarrow$	PaO_2 still low despite high F_1O_2 $PaCO_2$ normal.
	TRACHEOSTOMY LONGTERM IPPV $\downarrow$	
	WEANING EXTUBATION, RECOVERY	

tracheobronchitis or bronchopneumonia. Antibiotic treatment is determined by drug sensitivities to pathogenic organisms in the sputum. Occasionally it is necessary to start treatment before this information is available and then previous knowledge of the bacterial state of the burned skin is helpful in deciding which is the drug of choice. Additional respiratory support should be instituted if the clinical condition warrants it.

Adult Respiratory Distress Syndrome (ARDS)

This is a condition of respiratory failure with low PaO_2 despite oxygen administration, increased respiratory rate and tachycardia, which may occur in patients with or without a respiratory burn. It consists of persistent pulmonary oedema, the formation of hyaline membrane, and ultimately interstitial pulmonary fibrosis. Because of the multiple conditions that have been implicated in its aetiology, it is known by several other names, e.g. Shock lung, wet lung, respirator lung, stiff lung. Probably all these conditions are part of the same syndrome. The mortality of patients with established ARDS is high especially if associated with failure of other organs.

Possible causes of ARDS

1 Sepsis, e.g. associated with skin burns.
2 Prolonged hypotension, e.g. following inadequate resuscitation.
3 Respiratory burns, e.g. smoke, gas or acid inhalation. Loss of surfactant.
4 Massive blood transfusion especially of unfiltered blood, with micro-aggregates causing multiple micro-emboli in the lungs.
5 Micro-thrombosis due to diffuse intravascular coagulation (DIC) which may also be associated with massive blood transfusion.
6 Oxygen toxicity. IPPV with high oxygen concentrations may lead to the formation of hyaline membrane with subsequent failure of gaseous exchange. Therefore concentrations of inspired oxygen should not exceed 50%.

Effect of Low Serum Albumin

This may be low in burned patients because of loss of protein-rich fluid in blisters and oedema. If this has been inadequately replaced a low oncotic pressure may result. If this is lower than the pulmonary artery wedge pressure (measured with a Swann–Ganz catheter), there will be a transudation of fluid in the lungs. The treatment for this type of pulmonary oedema is an infusion of Plasma Protein Fraction (PPF).

Information from additional investigations

Chest X-ray

This may not show any abnormalities soon after a respiratory burn and serial studies may be required to demonstrate abnormal findings developing later.

Blood Gas Investigation (Table 16.3)

This is the measurement of the tension of oxygen and carbon dioxide in arterial blood. Most machines also measure pH and calculate bicarbonate automatically. Additional information, such as base excess may also be given.

Table 16.3   Information obtained by blood gas investigation

	Acidosis	Alkalosis
Respiratory	pH ↓	pH ↑
	$PaCO_2$ ↑	$PaCO_2$ ↓
		→HCO_3 ↓
	(Alveolar hypoventilation)	(Hyperventilation)
Metabolic	pH ↓	pH ↑
	HCO_3 ↓	(due to vomiting and diarrhoea and loss of Cl^-)
	(due to hypoxaemia)	
	→$PaCO_2$ ↓	HCO_3 ↑
		($PaCO_2$ ↑)

Method

Blood is commonly taken from the femoral, brachial or radial arteries. If frequent samples are required, the radial artery may be cannulated, although in burned patients, this may be considered undesirable due to the increased infection risk. The sample is taken into a 5 ml syringe, the dead space of which is filled with heparin. The sample is analysed immediately (and stored in ice in transit). The respiratory state of the patient at the time of sampling and the inspired oxygen concentration should be noted.

Information given

Oxygen. PaO_2 measures tension of oxygen in solution. Normally 0.3 ml of oxygen is carried in solution and 20 ml of oxygen is carried in combination with haemoglobin, per 100 ml of blood.

Normal value, breathing room air = 12–13 kPa.

Carbon dioxide. CO_2 is carried as bicarbonate, carbonic acid and carbamino-haemoglobin. The tension of CO_2 is dependent on the carbonic acid element (i.e. CO_2 in solution). $PaCO_2$ is the best measure of alveolar ventilation.

Normal value = 4.7–6.0 kPa.

pH. This is an expression of the hydrogen ion concentration (as a negative logarithm to base 10) and measures the acidity or alkalinity of the blood.

Normal value: 7.35–7.45.

Total bicarbonate. The sum of the bicarbonates of sodium, potassium, calcium and magnesium is usually calculated automatically.

Normal value 22–30 mmol/l.

Base excess. This is the surplus base or acid (base deficit is expressed as negative base excess) required to titrate the blood to pH 7.4 at $PaCO_2$ 5.3 kPa and 38°C.

Normal value = 2.5 ± 2.5 mmol/l.

For correction of metabolic acidosis, a simple formula can be used to calculate the amount of sodium bicarbonate needed:

Dose of bicarbonate in mmol =
    base deficit × 0.3 × bodyweight in kg.
2.74% solution of $NaHCO_3$ contains 166 mmol/500 ml
8.4%   solution of $NaHCO_3$ contains 1 mmol/ml.

Fibreoptic Bronchosocopy

This is most easily performed under general anaesthetic at the time of intubation or via an endotracheal tube. It gives direct visual evidence of the effect of the respiratory injury on the trachea and major bronchi. It is the most helpful early investigation.

Central Venous Pressure Measurement

This valuable measurement is not used routinely in burned patients because of the infection risk of a central line and the scarcity of veins in patients with large skin burns. However, it is very useful in patients who present particular haemodynamic problems, e.g. heart failure, septicaemic shock. During hypovolaemic shock, excessive blood loss and massive transfusion, CVP measurement gives an indication of adequacy of replacement and an early warning of overloading.

During IPPV, values are usually about 5 cm higher than during spontaneous respiration.

Normal value: 0–5 cm H_2O (above the level of the right atrium).

Swan–Ganz Catheterization

CVP measurement is a poor indicator of the state of the circulation in patients in whom there is an imbalance between right and left ventricular function, as a result of pre-existing or intercurrent heart or lung disease. For example, further clarification is required in the assessment of a patient with raised CVP, low BP and low urine output and co-existing left ventricular failure (from myocardial infarction) or right ventricular failure from increased pulmonary vascular resistance (from pulmonary emboli).

Further information is acquired by the technique of SG catheterization. A balloon-tipped catheter is inserted via a CVP approach and passed into the right atrium where the balloon is inflated. The catheter tip is then carried into the pulmonary artery in the blood flow. The position is checked by pressure measurements and X-ray. Most SG catheters wedge in the right lower lobe pulmonary artery.

Measurements of pressure, blood gases and temperature are taken and give the following information:

1 *Mixed venous PO₂*: Normal value: 5.3 kPa. This is a measure of tissue hypoxia as it shows the oxygen uptake by the tissues.
2 *Pressure measurements.*
   (a) CVP (right atrial pressure) Normal value 1–10 mmHg.
   (b) Pulmonary artery pressure. Normal value: $\dfrac{15-30}{5-12}$ mmHg.
   (c) Pulmonary artery wedge pressure (PAWP) Normal value: 5–15 mmHg. This is an index of left atrial pressure. This measurement may be useful in patients with ARDS, low serum albumin or left ventricular failure. Raised PAWP may indicate the need for inotropic support (dopamine).
3 *Cardiac output.* Normal value 5 l/min. This can be measured by a thermodilution method. A measured volume of cold saline is injected into the pulmonary artery and its dilution, as measured by a thermistor in the catheter tip, is estimated. A minicomputer presents the data as cardiac output. This measurement is useful in the monitoring of treatment with infusions or inotropic drugs.

References

BARTLETT, R.H. (1979) Respiratory Injury. *J. Trauma,* **19,** Suppl. 11, 918.

BARTLETT, R.H., NICCOLE, M., TAVIS, M.J., ALLYN, P.A. & FURNAS, D.W. (1976) Acute Management of the Upper Airway in Facial Burns and Smoke Inhalation. *Arch. Surg.,* **111,** 744.

BROWN, J.M. (1977) Inhalation Injury and Progressive Pulmonary Insufficiency. *Burns,* **4,** 32.

DESAI, M.H. (1984) Inhalation Injuries in Burn Victims. *Critical Care Quart.,* **7,** 1.

FLENLEY, D.C. (1978) Clinical Interpretation of Blood Gas and Acid-base Data. *B. J. Hosp. Med.,* **204,** 384.

HOROVITZ, J.H. (1979) Smoke Inhalation. *J. Trauma,* **19,** Supple. 11, 915.

HUNT, J.L., AGEE, R.N. & PRUITT, B.A. (1975) Fibreoptic Bronchoscopy in Acute Inhalation Injury. *J. Trauma,* **15,** 641.

KOHLER, G., BOCK, R., STRITZINGER, R., WEGENER, K. *et al.* (1981) Respiratory Complication Following Severe Burns – Pathological Findings. *Burns,* **8,** 123.

O'YA, H. (1976) Inhalation Burn; Statistical Study from Burns in Japan. *Burns,* **2,** 115.

SEVITT, S. (1974) *Reaction to Injury and Burns.* Wm. Heinemann, London.

VIVORI, E. & CUDMORE, R.E. (1977) Management of Airway Complications in Burned Children. *Br. Med. J.,* **2,** 1462.

ZAWACKI, B.E., JUNG, R.C., JOYCE, J. & RINCON, E. (1977) Smoke, Burns and the Natural History of Inhalation Injury in Fire Victims. *Ann. Surg.,* **185,** 100.

ZIKRIA, B.A. (1972) Smoke and Carbon Monoxide Poisoning. *J. Trauma,* **12,** 641.

17

Acute Renal Failure

Renal failure is diagnosed when the urine has
1 a fixed osmolality of 300–350 mOsm/kg H_2O
2 a specific gravity fixed at 1.010
3 urine urea to blood urea ratio of less than 10.

Oliguria is defined, in adults, as a urine output of less than 400 ml/ 24 hours. But urine volumes dropping below amounts shown on page 144 should be acted upon before such a low output occurs, for the solute load to be excreted requires a urine output of not less than about 5.5 ml/kg body weight/hour. Oliguria *per se* is not a reliable indication of renal failure; high-output failure is equally ominous.

Causes of poor urine output include:
1 Prerenal
  (a) Circulating volume depletion:
        Dehydration (usually due to delay in initiating adequate IV fluid replacement beyond about 2 hours post-burn).
        Loss into the extravascular space
        Blood Loss
  (b) Hypotension:
        Septic
        Cardiogenic
  (c) Vascular:
        Renal artery stenosis or vein thrombosis.
2 Post-renal:
  (a) Obstruction of outflow tract:
        Clot, trauma, calculus, tumour
        Prostatic hypertrophy or stricture
  (b) Bladder, ureteric or urethral rupture
  (c) Blocked catheter. Catheter not in bladder.
3 Renal
  (a) Acute tubular necrosis due to shock
  (b) Myoglobinuria, Haemoglobinuria
  (c) Nephrotoxicity (poisons, drugs)
  (d) Acute glomerular nephritis
  (e) Mismatched blood transfusion

Satisfactory urine outputs:
Children: 0 to   1 years: 10–20 ml/hour
              1 to 10 years: 20–30 ml/hour
            10 to 15 years: 25–35 ml/hour
Adults: 35–60 ml/hour
  or 0.5–1.0 ml/kg body weight/hour

Prevention of Renal Failure

It cannot be over-emphasized that prompt initiation of adequate intravenous fluid replacement within an hour or two at most of the burn injury will prevent the onset of many instances of renal failure.

Once reduced urine volumes are occurring, some cases can be reversed by making up the fluid volume which has been denied, by transfusing the amount due in the post-burn period which has been reached, plus the amount which should have been infused in the preceding periods (see page 45).

Inadequacy of circulating blood volume can be estimated by:
1 A consideration of the fluid input charts to date
2 Hourly urine output
3 Skin turgor
4 Haematocrit (haemoconcentration or haemodilution)
5 Jugular venous distension (when patient is supine, the jugular vein is usually visible up to the level of the posterior border of sternomastoid in thin people)
6 Urinary response to an IV fluid bolus challenge
7 Postural change in blood pressure (if measurable). The systolic and diastolic blood pressure should not drop more than 20 mmHg when the patient is sat up from lying.
8 Central venous (right atrial) pressure
9 Swan–Ganz (left atrial) pressure

Invasive catheterization is to be avoided if possible because of the danger of introducing septicaemia.

Haemoglobinuria and Myoglobinuria (Fig. 7.1, p.45)

Haemoglobinuria, recognized by black urine passing in the urinary catheter, results from the lysis of red cells which become fragile following burn injury. Some red cells are probably also damaged at the site of deep heat injury. Provided the haemoglobinuria can be cleared within 24 hours renal failure usually does not occur, but persistence beyond 24 hours is increasingly ominous. Myoglobinuria from crushed or necrotic muscle produces similar complications.

A diuresis with 1 g mannitol/kg body weight in a 20% solution, intravenously, may result in elimination of the haemoglobin, but a careful watch must be kept for the onset of pulmonary oedema.

Established Renal Failure

Once renal failure is threatened (see page 143) a nephrologist should be brought into the management.

This point, for practical purposes, has probably been reached when a least one of the following is observed:

1 Rate of rise in serum creatinine is above 1.6 mg/100 ml/24 hours (140 μmol/litre/24 hours).
2 Rate of rise in blood urea nitrogen above 28.0 mg/100 ml/24 hours (4.7 mmol/litre/24 hours).
3 Blood urea rising above 200 mg/100 ml (34 mmol/l).
4 Serum potassium rising above 7.0 mmol/l and unresponsive to measures detailed below.
5 Urine volume falling below 250 ml/24 hours for 3 days.

Management

1 Treatment of the cause if known, e.g. excision of crushed muscle, of septicaemia, drainage of pus etc.
2 Hyperkalaemia. Calcium resonium 15–30 g two to four times daily orally or as a retention enema should be started when the serum potassium reaches 6 mmol/l, M/6 sodium lactate 450 ml with 50 ml of 50% dextrose IV over two or three hours. Half an hour after start of the infusion, 10 units of soluble insulin IV. This regime may be repeated once only, and is started as soon as the ECG shows peaking of the T wave or the serum potassium reaches 7 mmol/l.

    Further deterioration in the ECG (i.e. widening of the QRS complex) requires intravenous calcium in sufficient quantity to reverse the changes. Dialysis should be urgently considered.
3 Metabolic acidosis, controlled with sodium bicarbonate, but beware hypernatraemia. Slow rising acidosis may not need correction.
4 Anaemia, by infusion of packed cells (if fluid volume is adequate) or whole blood.

Diet

Protein 0.5–1 g/kg body weight/day
Potassium 2 g/day
Sodium 2 g/day
Fluid: Insensible losses (500–800 ml/day) plus measured urine
output, diarrhoea and vomitus plus 200 ml/one degree of
temperature over 38°C per day
Calories: as in Sutherland and Batchelor charts (page 159)
Vitamins

Drugs

Avoid:
  Tetracycline
  Nitrofurantoin
  Nalidixic acid
Avoid if possible:
  Aminoglycosides (gentamycin, tobramycin, amikacin)
  Carbenicillin
  Kanamycin
  Neomycin
  Streptomycin
  Vancomycin
  Dextran

Urine Catheter

If anuric, consider intermittent catheterization (i.e. once daily) rather
than risking pyocystus (pus in the bladder) with an indwelling
catheter.

Haemodialysis

Details of haemodialysis are outside the scope of this book. They
will be given by the nephrologist. The surgeon may however be
expected to provide vascular access and some consideration of these
techniques is therefore included.

Dialysis Equipment

The characteristics of the semi-permeable membrane which separates the patient's blood from the dialysate fluid determines the composition of the dialysate fluid, the rates of flow and the filtration rates.

Blood is usually removed from the patient via a roller pump from an artery, vein, shunt or fistula. Since this line contains a negative pressure, it is advisable to have a drip chamber or other means of ensuring that bubbles do not enter the dialyser where they would compromise the transfer of solutes.

Similarly, a drip chamber is incorporated on the line returning blood to the patient. A positive pressure is required in this delivery line.

Vascular Access

Percutaneous dialysis catheter

The femoral or subclavian veins may be used. To provide the line to remove blood from the patient:
1 A 16-gauge cannula is inserted into the femoral vein and a Seldinger spring guidewire introduced through it up to the iliac vein for 15–20 cm;
2 The cannula is withdrawn;
3 A Teflon catheter is slid over the guidewire up to the inferior vena cava;
4 The guidewire is removed;
5 Using a Luer-Lock fitting, the dialysis tubing is fixed to the Teflon catheter.
6 1000 units heparin in 500 ml saline is continuously infused at 5 ml/ hour.

The venous line to return blood to the patient is provided by cannulating a peripheral vein with a 16 gauge catheter or using a double lumen coaxial catheter in the inferior vena cava.

Complications include: iliofemoral vein thrombosis; retroperitoneal haemorrhage; infection at the catheter site.

Scribner shunt

The usual site is the distal forearm using the radial artery and cephalic vein, but other vessels, not necessarily anatomically adjacent, may be used if circumstances demand. It is advisable not to use vessels near joints. As with other methods, the usable sites will be determined by those areas away from burned tissue.
1 Two Silastic tubes each with a tapered Teflon tip are introduced, one each into artery and vein, via skin incisions.
2 The vessels are encircled with 4-0 silk proximally and distally.
3 The distal sutures are tied, leaving the ends long.

4 Through an arteriotomy or venotomy, the Teflon catheter is advanced proximally into the artery and the vein, beyond the proximal ligature.
5 The proximal suture is tied, holding the catheter.
6 The long ends of the distal suture are tied over the catheter, fixing it against the vessel.
7 The long ends of the proximal and the distal sutures are tied to each other, to prevent the vessel pulling apart.
8 The arterial and venous catheters may be joined with a connector.

Complications of Haemodialysis

1 Hypotension: When removal of fluid from the patient is too rapid hypotension ensues.
2 Hypertension: Though less usual, this may result when renin is released.
3 Convulsions: More frequent in children than in adults, the too rapid removal of urea may cause fitting.
4 Fever, headache, backache, shivering may be due to:
   (a) a blood transfusion reaction;
   (b) reaction to the materials in the dialysis machine, or contamination.
5 Bleeding: Gastrointestinal, retroperitoneal, pericardial bleeding may result from the heparinization.
6 Hypoventilation: Oxygen by mask is usually sufficient to overcome this effect which occurs chiefly in patients with marginal pulmonary sufficiency before dialysis.
7 Air embolus: Since the arterial line is under negative pressure, the addition of drugs and fluids into this line must be carried out with extreme care.

Peritoneal Dialysis

Indications for Peritoneal Dialysis

Relative indications for preferring peritoneal instead of haemodialysis include:
1 Patients with cardiac instability (arrhythmia)
2 Patients with labile blood pressures or hypertension
3 Patients in whom suitable vessel access is unavailable
4 When heparin is contraindicated because of acute haemorrhage
   Peritoneal dialysis is more widely available than haemodialysis, and, although less adequate clearances are produced it provides a

more even control of hyperkalaemia than does intermittent haemodialysis. When repeated peritoneal dialysis is anticipated, the Tenckhoff catheter is suitable. Each treatment takes up to 12 hours, and may be repeated daily or three times weekly. It is desirable that the lower abdomen is unburned.

The bladder is emptied by catheter.

The lower abdominal skin is thoroughly cleansed with antiseptic.

The skin 5 cm (2 in) below the umbilicus is infiltrated with local anaesthetic, and a 0.5 cm skin incision made with a scalpel. The catheter is introduced in the midline into the peritoneal space, and connected to a closed system with a 3-way tap for introduction of the dialysis fluid and for drainage. Dialysis fluid warmed to 37°C is run into the peritoneal cavity.

Accurate records of input and drainage volumes are maintained.

Complications

1 Abdominal pain probably indicates the fluid is being run in too rapidly or under too high a pressure
2 Peritonitis. Return of a murky fluid, abdominal pain and fever necessitate bacteriological culture of a sample. An antibiotic is added to the dialysis fluid. Peritoneal dialysis may have to be discontinued if symptoms and signs cannot be controlled.
3 Blockage. Should the input exceed the volume which drains, omentum may have wrapped around the catheter. This may be dislodged by giving caster oil 5 to 20 ml orally. More usually the catheter needs to be resited.

References

BELL, P. R. F. & WOOD, R. F. M. (1983) *Surgical Aspects of Haemodialysis.* 2nd ed, Churchill Livingstone, Edinburgh.

BRENNER, B. M. & SKEIN, J. H. (1980) *Acute Renal Failure.* Churchill Livingstone, Edinburgh.

BRUNS, D. E., HEROLD, D. A., RODEHEAVER, G. T. & EDLICH, R. F. (1982) Polyethylene Glycol Intoxication in Burn Patients. *Burns, 9,* 49.

DAVISON, A. M. (1978) *Dialysis Review.* Pitman Medical, London.

POMERANZ, A., REICHBERG, Y. et al. (1985) Peritoneal Dialysis in a Burned Patient. *Burns, 11,* 367.

SAWADA, Y., MOMMA, S. et al. (1984) Survival from Acute Renal Failure after Severe Burns. *Burns, 11,* 143.

SETTLE, J. A. (1975) Urine Output following Severe Burns. *Burns, 1,* 23.

SEVITT, S. (1974) *Reactions to Injury and Burns.* Heinemann, London.

TILNEY, N. L. & LAZARUS, J. M. (1982) *Surgical Care of the Patient with Renal Failure.* W. B. Saunders, Philadelphia.

18

Special Considerations in Nursing Paediatric Burn Patients

Approximately 50% of all major burn victims are children. This is partly due to children being more prone to accidental injury, but also to the fact that children have a larger body surface area in proportion to body weight than adults. Since it is surface area burned that largely decrees the severity of the burn illness, the child will be more acutely affected by what might appear a relatively minor burn in an adult (see Chapter 5, p.29).

Ideally children should be cared for in a paediatric unit where all the staff are experienced in caring for children. In practice there are very few specialized Paediatric Burns Units, therefore child victims of major burn injury are more commonly cared for in burns units which cater for all ages and have some members of the burn care team who are paediatric specialists. Consequently experienced 'burns team' members also become very experienced in paediatric care.

The care of a child with burns differs from that of an adult because of:
1 Different physical responses and needs.
2 Decreased co-operation.
3 Increased psychological trauma.
4 Different emotional needs (according to his stage of development).
5 Different nutritional needs.
6 Different cosmetic needs.
7 The needs of his parents and family.
8 The child is more prone to complications.

150

Different Physical Responses and Needs

Compared to an adult the head and trunk of a child are larger in proportion to the rest of his body, and the body surface of a child younger than 10 years is larger in proportion to body weight than in an adult. Therefore a different chart is required for estimating percentage surface area burned, (see Lund and Bowder Chart page 29).

The child's physical response to hypo- or hypervolaemia is likely to fluctuate more than an adult. Therefore great care is required in control of input and accurate measurement of output. An electronic drip regulator is probably the safest method of controlling fluid intake, but if this is not available a burette must be fitted to the delivery set and monitored continuously.

Wound infection, which may convert the burn wound from partial thickness into full thickness skin loss, is more likely in children than adults. Therefore, despite the undesirable emotional effects of isolation, it may be necessary to protect himself and/or others.

Children's response to drugs is very different from that of adults and the nurse must be familiar with paediatric formulae, methods of administration and likely complications.

Decreased Co-operation

The degree to which a child is able to co-operate depends on the child's age and stage of development.

If the nurse understands the normal development of the child she can estimate the likely response to the various nursing procedures and help the child to co-operate. For example:

Infants can easily be distracted so that their attention is focused away from an unpleasant procedure.

Toddlers are trying to establish their identity and are liable to do the opposite of what is asked. Playful teasing like 'I don't want you to have that delicious drink, I'm going to drink it' may persuade a reluctant child to drink.

Older children may respond well to reasoned explanation geared to their level of understanding.

Confrontation is avoided by withdrawing from the situation and trying a different approach later.

The burned child is highly likely to require future admission for reconstructive surgery, therefore the importance of gaining his co-operation and trust cannot be overstressed. No child should be forced into submission unless the treatment to be given is life saving. There are many ways of persuading a child to co-operate and each must be tried until success is achieved.

Increased Psychological Trauma

A severe burn injury, the resulting critical illness, and the change in body image due to scarring, are very harrowing experiences at any age, but are likely to be more so in a child who does not understand and is not capable of reasoned thought. In addition any admission to hospital can be a traumatic experience for a child which may have serious consequences for the child and his family for many years.

First impressions are very important even to an infant or critically ill child. The admission room for a child should be suitably prepared to please and entertain him as much as possible.

Pictures and 'mobiles' will attract an infant's attention and stimulate his natural curiosity in his environment.

The toddler will be stimulated and helped to communicate by soft toys and picture books.

The parents are encouraged to bring to the hospital any special or favourite toys, which can be a great source of comfort to the child. Some concern has been expressed about bringing 'dirty' toys into the 'clean' environment of a burns unit or intensive care unit, but there is no evidence that such toys are a source of infection.

The older child needs a television, access to a telephone and an ample supply of books and games (probably in that order of priority).

The degree of psychological trauma experienced by the child is influenced by:
1 The age of the child.
2 The child/parent relationship.
3 Any previous experience of separation.
4 The severity of the burn illness and consequent scarring.
5 The quality of the care given while in hospital.
6 After-care given following the child's discharge from hospital.

At a time when a child is subjected to a large team of strangers, who make various demands of him, it is vital that he gains confidence and trust in his 'carers'. One nurse is assigned to the child to act as his special friend and, where necessary, as surrogate parent. It is important that all members of the team know and understand the 'unique' role of this nurse to the child.

The whole team co-ordinate their efforts to assist the child through his 'special' nurse, who acts for the child as his protector, go-between and if the child is old enough, his negotiator.

The child's 'special nurse' should not actively participate in any unpleasant or painful procedure. Her role is to comfort and reassure the child that the outcome will be optimistic, and to retain his trust in her.

Different Emotional Needs

To understand the different emotional needs of a child the nurse must have a clear understanding of normal child development at all ages.

The nurse gleans from the parents as much information as possible about the child;

his stage of development,

his personality,

any particular likes and dislikes,

any particular fears or anxieties,

how the parents normally interact with, manage and discipline the child,

his favourite toys, TV programmes, hobbies.

The nurse also learns from the parents their own views and desires regarding their child's care and, wherever possible, ensures that their beliefs and requests are respected by all members of the team.

The child's parents are encouraged to participate in his care as much as possible and to take part in any discussion and decision making related to the child's care. It is particularly important for the infant and young child that his mother be encouraged to remain with him throughout his hospitalization, and adequate accommodation and facilities for parents are a vital part of any paediatric intensive care area.

It is essential to the young child's development that he be picked up, cuddled and spoken to irrespective of dressings, splintage and attachment to machines. The nurse must gain the parent's confidence and ensure that they have been adequately reassured that they will not harm the child by cuddling him in spite of the equipment and attachments surrounding him, so that they do not communicate any fear or nervousness to their child.

In addition to caring for the child's immediate and obvious emotional needs the nurse ensures that he has adequate stimulation and encouragement through play and education to continue his normal development.

Different Nutritional Needs

The special nutritional needs of burn victims are discussed in Chapter 19. The nutritional needs of the burnt child vary according to age, weight and body surface area burnt (see chart page 159).

As with adults, inadequate nutrition in the burnt child delays wound healing and predisposes the child to infection. The child may in addition suffere delay in physical development.

Maintaining adequate nutrition in the critically ill child is hampered by the child's natural loss of appetite and lack of comprehension of the importance of good nutrition. In addition he is prone to vomit due to anxiety and emotional distress, forced feeding with a diet of which he is unfamiliar, and paralytic ileus resulting from the stress of the burn illness.

The child's normal dietary history is carefully documented, including any particular likes and dislikes. The diet plan is then tailor-made for each child ensuring that his 'special likes' are incorporated into his daily nutritional requirements.

The parents are encouraged to accompany the child at meal times to encourage him, but care must be taken not to make the parents over-anxious regarding their child's intake as this may only increase the child's anxiety and lead to additional feeding problems. For the reluctant toddler there are may aids to encourage drinking and eating, such as comic mugs and trick straws.

Naso-gastric tube feeding should be used only as a last resort for children, but may be life saving for the critically ill child who is unable or unwilling to take his nutritional requirements orally.

Different Cosmetic Needs

The child's body image is different from an adult, depending on his mental age and development.

The infant learns to differentiate his own body from his surroundings by sensation and self exploration. The stimulation necessary for this development is hampered by burn dressings and splints. To compensate for this the child is cuddled, rocked and stroked to provide the essential stimulation.

The toddler (1–3 years) is learning to differentiate self from environment, and struggling to exert his autonomy. He may experience difficulty in defining his body boundaries and may see burn dressings as a part of himself. Play is directed at helping the child to seek out and understand his own body limits.

The pre-school child (3–5 years) understands his body boundaries and is beginning to identify with the parent, to develop sexual curiosity, and conform to sex-typing. The attitude of the parents has the most marked effect on the child at this stage in helping him form a 'good' self image.

The school aged child has to compete with peers. Acceptance by his friends is essential at this stage of development. The child who is disfigured and possibly physically disabled by his burn needs constant encouragement and praise for his achievements to encourage a healthy self image. Initially competition with other disfigured or disabled children will improve the child's body image and for this purpose self help groups can be very useful.

The adolescent is undergoing many bodily changes related to sexual development. He tends to be self conscious and over-anxious about his appearance. Consequently much time and effort are required to counsel the burnt adolescent to ensure that he adapts to his changed body image and does not overemphasize his defects.

The Needs of the Parents and Family

Caring for the parents and family is an essential part of caring for a child. In addition to their distress and anxiety at the severity of their child's illness and the appearance of his wounds the parents often feel guilty, probably because of a sense of failure to protect the child from harm. Parents also frequently display feelings of anger, often directed toward one another if one blames the other for the accident.

Obviously such emotional problems in the parents can only be harmful for the child's psychological care, therefore as much time as is necessary must be spent on counselling the parents and family to help them understand and overcome their own feelings.

Encouraging the parents to participate in caring for their child and helping in making the decisions regarding his care will enable them to overcome feelings of guilt, anger and rejection.

Even where the accident was clearly preventable it is not helpful to the child's wellbeing if the nurse displays her own feelings of anger toward the parents.

Non-accidental Injury

The nurse must be constantly alert for the signs of child abuse, and ensure immediate and effective action in all suspected cases.

The evidence the nurse may be able to supply may be vital information in deciding the future care of the child. For example:

The child's story as to the cause of the accident compared to the way the parents related it.

The child's reaction to and interaction with his parents.

The parents' interaction with each other.

The immediate appearance of the burn, whether or not the appearance fits the description of the accident.

Any unexplained fears and anxieties in the child.

All such information should be carefully and accurately documented to ensure that evidence does not become distorted with the passage of time and further experience of the child, parents and family.

Although it is essential to identify all cases of child abuse, it is equally important that parents are not wrongly accused, as the added anxiety this causes may result in rejection of the child and so jeopardize his future.

Paediatric Dosage

Young's formula:

$$\text{Child's dose} = \frac{\text{Age of child (years)}}{\text{Age of child} + 12} \times \text{Adult dose}$$

Clark's formula:

$$\text{Child's dose} = \frac{\text{Wt. of child (kg)}}{70} \times \text{Adult dose}$$

References

BOTTOMLEY, E.(1981) *Thermal Injury in Children*. Medical Education (International) Ltd.

BOWDEN, M. L. & FELLER, I.(1973) Family Reaction to a Severe Burn. *Am. J. Nursing*, **73**, 317.

DEWET, B., CYWES, S. *et al.* (1979) Aspects of Post Treatment Adjustment in Burned Children. *Burns*, **5**, 321.

DUNCOMBE, M. & WELLER, B. S.(1979) *Paediatric Nursing*. Baillière Tindall, London.

FOWLER, J.(1979) Parent Groups in Rehabilitation of the Burned Child. *Burns*, **5**, 86.

GILJOHANN, A.(1981) Adolescents Burned as Children. *Burns*, **7**, 95.

MARTIN, H.(1981) Psychological Effects of Accidental Injury in Childhood. *Burns*, **7**, 90.

MARTIN, H.(1970) Parents and Children's Reactions to Burns and Scalds. *Br. J. Med. Psychol.*, **43**, 183.

MURRAY CLARKE, A. & MARTIN, H. L. (1979) Effects of Previous Thermal Injury on Adolescents. *Burns*, **5**, 101.

POTTER, J. & CLAUDE, P. R.(1970) Characteristics of Burned Children after Injury. *Br. J. Plastic Surg.*, **23**, 63.

QUINBY, S. & BERNSTEIN, N.(1971) How Children Live after Disfiguring Burns. *Psychiat. Med.*, **2**, 146.

SAWYER, M. G., MINDE, K. & ZUKER, R.(1983) The Burned Child. *Burns*, **9**, 205.

WAGNER, M. M.(1981) *Care of the Burn Injured Patient*. Croom Helm, London.

WILKINS, T. J. & CAMPBELL, J. L.(1981) Psychosocial Concerns in a Paediatric Burn Unit. *Burns*, **7**, 208.

WOODWARD, J.(1959) Emotional Disturbances of Burned Children. *Br. Med. J.*, **1**, 1009.

WRIGHT, L. & FULWILER, R.(1974) Longrange Emotional Sequelae of Burns. *Pediatr. Res.*, **8**, 931.

YIACOUMETTIS, A. & ROBERTS, M.(1975) Analysis of Burns in Children. *Burns*, **3**, 195.

19

Nutrition in Burns

Modern burn care has been significantly improved by the better understanding of nutritional requirements, improvement in estimating requirements and the provision of methods of feeding that are more comfortable for the patient and convenient to prepare and administer.

Hence the dietician has become an indispensable member of the burn care team, being responsible for the provision of tailor-made feeds for each patient, monitoring the patient's intake daily and adjusting his diet to provide accurate amounts of calories, nitrogen, vitamins and essential elements to correct any deficiencies.

Immediately after the burn injury metabolism enters a catabolic phase which lasts for up to 5 days. If there is infection the catabolic phase will persist until the infection is eradicated. This catabolism causes:

1 Increase in loss of protein;
2 Urinary excretion of nitrogen is increased by up to 300%;
3 Rapid loss of weight as muscle protein is broken down and converted into glucose to provide energy;
4 Some of this glucose may be excreted in the urine (glycosuria).

To add to the problems created by the catabolic state the energy needs following burn injury are increased.

Therefore the total nutritional needs of the patient may amount to 2 or 3 times his normal intake. An adult weighing 60 kg with a 60% burn requires 5400 kcal plus 38.4 g of nitrogen daily. The burn patient is therefore unlikely to be able to eat the quantities of natural food necessary to provide all his requirements.

To provide adequate nutrition it is essential to establish a high calorie, high protein intake from the third post-burn day at the latest. The natural loss of appetite following any major burn injury adds to the patient's difficulty in taking his nutritional needs.

Meals must be carefully compiled, prepared and presented to provide the required nutrition in the form the patient will find most appetizing and palatable. The dietician explains to the patient, or for a young child to his parents, his dietary needs resulting from the burn injury, and finds out what type of diet the patient is used to, what foods he particularly likes and dislikes, and how much he usually eats each day. His feeds are then prepared to provide the necessary daily requirement as shown in the Sutherland and Batchelor Charts (Table 19.1).

Table 19.1 Burns nutrition: Table of energy requirements (kcal) and nitrogen requirements (g) (in parentheses) per day.

Weight kg	*Percentage of body surface burned*			
	20%	40%	60%	80%
Adults				
40	2200 (16.0)	3600 (25.6)	5000 (35.2)	6400 (44.8)
60	2600 (19.2)	4000 (28.8)	5400 (38.4)	6800 (48.0)
70	2800 (20.8)	4200 (30.4)	5600 (40.0)	7000 (49.6)
90	3200 (24.0)	4600 (33.6)	6000 (43.2)	7400 (52.8)
100	3400 (25.6)	4800 (35.2)	6200 (44.8)	7600 (54.4)
Children				
5	1000 (5.6)	1000 (5.6)	1000 (5.6)	1000 (5.6)
10	1300 (8.0)	1300 (8.0)	1300 (8.0)	1300 (8.0)
15	1600 (10.4)	1950 (12.0)	1950 (12.0)	1950 (12.0)
20	1900 (12.8)	2600 (16.0)	3300 (19.2)	4000 (22.4)
30	2500 (17.6)	3200 (20.8)	3900 (24.0)	4600 (27.2)

Data adapted from Sutherland, A. B. and Batchelor, A. D. R. *Ann. N. Y. Acad. Sci.,* (1968), **150**, 700; and *Burns,* (1976), **2**, 238.

Appetizing meals of foods he particularly likes are given and the actual amounts eaten are carefully recorded. The daily deficit is then provided by supplementary feeds in the form of pleasant-tasting drinks, e.g. Express Standard, Ensure Plus.

If the quantity of fluid the supplementary feeds represent is too much for the patient to take orally, the balance is given by continuous slow intra-gastric drip via a narrow-bore nasogastric tube.

If the patient is unconscious or for any other reason unable to eat or drink, the entire daily nutritional requirements are given via the nasogastric tube.

Most patients are initially unable to tolerate the administration of the total daily nutritional requirements and develop diarrhoea and vomiting if full strength supplementary feeds are commenced on day one of the feeding regime. Therefore feeding is commenced with half-strength feeds and gradually increased to full strength over the next 3–7 days.

Full aseptic care is required in handling and administering feeds if contamination and the risks of diarrhoea (or, rarely, septicaemia) are to be avoided. If diarrhoea develops despite the gradual introduction of full-strength feeds, kaolin or codeine phosphate are administered rather than prolonging the failure to meet the patient's nutritional needs. A persistently low serum albumen or a weight loss of more than 10% of initial weight indicates that the patient is not receiving adequate nutrition, and is an ominous sign in burn victims.

The patient is weighed at least weekly to ensure that he is retaining as near his admission weight as possible. The feeding requirement is adjusted as the burn heals and the surface area of skin loss is reduced (as per Batchelor and Sutherland Chart). Supplementary feeding is continued until the patient is fully healed and has reached his admission weight. In practice most major burn victims are fully healed and ready for discharge home whilst still a few pounds short of their admission weight. Therefore, the importance of continued good nutritional control on discharge are explained to the patient and his family.

Table 19.2   Average weights and measures of common foods

Milk for 1 cup	30 g
1 glass	200 g
Cheese 1 inch cube	20 g
Steak (7 oz)	200 g
Bacon 1 rasher	30 g
Sausage	55 g
Egg (one)	55 g
Butter/margarine for 1 slice bread	6 g
Potato, one medium size	110 g
mashed, one scoop	55 g
Orange, one medium	100 g
Apple, one medium	80 g
Bread, 1 slice	30–60 g
Cornflakes, 1 helping	30 g
Biscuit	7 g
Coffee, one cup	2 g
Beer, 1 pint	570 ml
Wine, 1 glass	70 ml

Table 19.3   Composition of foods per 100 g or 3.6 oz. (Adapted from Manual of Nutrition ref book 342. Ministry of Agriculture, Fisheries & Food HMSO, 1981)

	Energy (kcal)	(k J)	Protein (g)	Fat (g)	Carbohydrate (g)
Dairy Products					
Milk, liquid	65	272	3	4	5
skimmed	34	142	3	0.1	5
Cream, single	195	806	2	19	3
Cheese, cheddar	406	1682	26	33	0
cottage	96	402	14	4	1
Eggs	147	612	12	11	0
Butter	740	3041	0	82	0
Margarine	730	3000	0	81	0

Table 19.3 *Continued*

	Energy (kcal)	(k J)	Protein (g)	Fat (g)	Carbohydrate (g)
Meat					
Cooked bacon rasher	447	1851	24	39	0
Corned beef	217	905	27	12	0
Roast chicken	142	599	26	4	0
Cooked ham	269	1119	25	19	0
Roast lamb	291	1209	23	22	0
Pork chop, grilled	332	1380	28	24	0
Pork sausage	367	1520	11	32	9
Beef sausage	299	1242	10	24	12
Fish					
White fish	76	322	17	1	0
Fried cod	199	834	20	10	7
Fish fingers	178	749	13	7	16
Preserves					
Jam	262	1116	0	0	69
Honey	288	1229	0	0	76
White sugar	394	1680	0	0	105
Vegetables					
Runner beans	24	102	2	0	4
Broad beans	69	293	7	0	9
Boiled brussels sprouts	18	75	3	0	2
Boiled cabbage	15	16	2	0	2
Cauliflower	13	56	2	0	1
Potato crisps	533	2224	6	36	49
Boiled peas, frozen	38	161	5	8	4
Canned peas	76	325	6	0	14
Potatoes, boiled	79	339	1.4	0	20
Chips, fried	253	1065	4	11	37
Potatoes, roast	157	662	3	5	27
Fruit					
Apple	46	196	0	0	12
Orange	35	150	1	0	8
Pear	41	175	0	0	11
Plum	32	137	1	0	8
Cereals					
Bread, brown	223	948	9	2	45
white	233	991	8	2	50
wholemeal	216	918	9	3	42
Cornflakes	368	1567	9	2	85
Biscuit, plain	457	1925	7	17	75
Rice	361	1536	6	1	87

Table 19.3   *Continued*

	Energy (kcal)	(k J)	Protein (g)	Fat (g)	Carbohydrate (g)
Beverages					
Chocolate, drinking	366	1554	5	6	77
Coffee, instant	100	424	15	0	11
Tea	0	0	0	0	0
Squash, fruit	122	521	0	0	32
Beer, keg	31	129	0	0	23
Spirits 70° proof	222	919	0	0	0
Wine, red	68	284	0	0	0
Soup, tomato, canned	55	230	1	3	6
Ice cream	166	698	3	7	23
Rice pudding	131	552	4	4	20

Table 19.4   Nutrition: Average minimum requirements

	Adults (per kg/24 hours)	Children (per kg/24 hours)
Fat	2 g	4 g
Carbohydrate	2–3 g	12–18 g
Protein	0.6–0.9 g	1.8 g
Energy	35–40 kcal	90–125 kcal
Water	30–35 ml	100–150 ml

200 kcals of carbohydrate are needed to utilize 1 g of Nitrogen

Calorific values

Fat	9.0 kcal/g	Protein	4.2 kcal/g
Carbohydrate	4.0 kcal/g	Alcohol	7.0 kcal/g
Nitrogen	0.67 kcal/g		

Loss of Nitrogen per day

is the sum of

1 Urine loss = 24 hour urine urea in mmol $\times \dfrac{3.38}{100}$

2 Blood urea correction = increase in blood urea in

$$\text{mmol/l} \times \text{wt(kg)} \times \dfrac{17.35}{1000}$$

3 Proteinuria loss = urine protein in g/24h $\times$ 0.16 gives the total loss in g of nitrogen.

   1 g of nitrogen = 6.25 g protein

Table 19.5 Nutrient composition of skimmed, semi-skimmed and full cream milk (per pint)

	Energy (kcal)	Protein (g)	Fat (g)	Carbohydrate (g)	Calcium (mg)	Iron (mg)	Vitamin 'A' (µg)	Thiamin (mg)	Riboflavin (mg)	Nicotinic Acid (mg)	Vitamin 'C' (mg)	Vitamin 'D' (µg)
Milk liquid, whole	380	19.3	22.2	27.5	702	0.3	228	0.23	1.11	5.03	6	0.13
Milk liquid, semi-skimmed	266	19.6	9.1	28.2	725	0.3	89	0.23	1.13	5.08	6	0.05
per 100 ml	46.8	3.4	1.6	4.9	127.6	0.05	15.6	0.04	0.19	0.89	1.0	0.008
Milk liquid, skimmed	193	19.9	0.6	29.3	761	0.3	Trace	0.23	1.17	5.15	6	Trace

Table 19.6 Enteral nutrition

	Quantity	k cal	kJoules	Protein (g)	Nitrogen (g)	Fat (g)	Carbohydrate	Presentation as an oral feed	Naso-gastric tube
Complete Feeds									
Clinifeed vanilla 400 (Roussel)	5 cans (each 375 ml)	2000	8360	75	12	67	275	Ready to use	Fine bore
Clinifeed protein-rich (Roussel)	4 cans	2000	8360	120	19	44	280	Ready to use	Fine bore
Complan (Glaxo)	450 g	1998	8311	90	14	72	248	Mix in water	Fine bore
Ensure (Abbots)	8 cans (each 235 ml)	2024	8464	70	11	70	275	Ready to use	Fine bore
Flexical (elemental) (Bristol-Myers)	450 g	2000	8360	45	7	68	304	Mix in water	Fine bore

Table 19.6 Enteral nutrition *continued*

	Quantity	k cal	kJoules	Protein (g)	Nitrogen (g)	Fat (g)	Carbohydrate	Presentation as an oral feed	Nasto-gastric tube
Galactomine Formula 17 (Cow & Gate)	400 g	1912	7950	88	14	88	200	Mix in water	Fine bore
Isocal (Bristol-Myers)	6 cans (each 355 ml)	2190	9162	73	12	94	280	Ready to use	Fine bore
Nutruaxil (KabiVitrum)	4 bottles (each 500 ml)	2000	8360	76	12	68	276	Ready to use	Fine bore
Trisorbon (Merck)	5 sachets (each 85 g)	2000	8360	80	13	80	238	Mix in water	Ryles tube
Vivonex HN (Norwich Eaton) (elemental)	7 sachets (each 80 g)	2100	8792	72	12	2	443	Mix in water	Fine bore
Nutritional Supplements									
Build-up (Carnation)	6 sachets (each 38 g)	1890	7902	108	17	72	228	Add 1 sachet to 280 ml (½pt) milk	Ryles tube
Caloreen (Roussel)	500 g	2000	8360	0	0	0	500	Add to food, fluids	
Maxipro HBV (Scientific Hosp. Supplies)	600 g	2112	8568	528	84	24	0	Sprinkle into food and mix in fluids in small quantities	
Prosparol (Duncan, Flockhart)	500 ml	2250	9405	0	0	250	0	Whip and mix into food and drinks	

NB. Many of the above are unsuitable for young children without additional fluids. Galactomine and other specialized baby feeds,

Table 19.7 Guidelines for body weight. Heights are without shoes. Weights are unclothed. (Adapted from *J. R. Coll. Phys. Lond.*, (1983) 17, 7.

Height		MEN				WOMEN			
		Average		Normal range		Average		Normal range	
Feet in	Metric (m)	Stones lbs	kg	Stones lbs	kg	Stones lbs	kg	Stones lbs	kg
4 10	1.48					7 4	46	6 8- 8 7	42–54
4 11	1.50					7 6	47	6 10- 8 10	43–55
5 0	1.52					7 9	48	6 12- 8 13	44–57
5 1	1.55					7 12	50	7 1- 9 2	44–58
5 2	1.58	8 11	56	8 0–10 1	51–64	8 1	51	7 4- 9 5	45–58
5 3	1.60	9 1	58	8 3–10 4	52–65	8 4	53	7 7- 9 8	48–61
5 4	1.63	9 4	59	8 6–10 8	54–67	8 8	55	7 10- 9 12	50–64
5 5	1.66	9 7	61	8 9–10 12	55–69	8 11	57	7 13–10 2	51–65
5 6	1.68	9 10	62	8 12–11 2	56–71	9 2	58	8 2–10 6	52–66
5 7	1.70	10 0	63	9 2–11 7	58–73	9 6	60	8 6–10 10	53–67
5 8	1.73	10 5	65	9 6–11 12	59–74	9 10	61	8 10–11 0	55–69
5 9	1.76	10 9	67	9 10–12 2	62–77	10 0	64	9 0–11 4	58–72
5 10	1.78	10 13	69	10 0–12 6	64–79	10 4	65	9 4–11 9	59–74
5 11	1.80	11 4	71	10 4–12 11	65–80	10 8	67	9 8–12 0	61–76
6 0	1.83	11 8	73	10 8–13 2	66–82	10 12	69	9 12–12 5	63–78
6 1	1.86	11 12	76	10 12–13 7	69–86				
6 2	1.88	12 3	78	11 2–13 12	71–88				
6 3	1.90	12 8	79	11 6–14 3	73–90				
6 4	1.93	12 13	81	11 10–14 8	75–93				

References

AULICK, L. H., HANDER, E. W.*et al.* (1979) Thermal and Metabolic Demands on Burns Hypermetabolism. *J. Trauma,* **19**, 559.

BINGHAM, H. G., KRISCHER, J. P., SHUSTER, J. J. & ENGELMAN, I. E.(1980) Effects of Nutrition on Length of Stay and Survival for Burned Patients. *Burns,* **7**, 252.

CURRIERI, P. W.(1975) Metabolic and Nutritional Aspects of Thermal Injury. *Burns,* **2**, 16.

CURRIERI, P. W.(1979) Nutritional Replacement Modalities. *J. Trauma,* **19**, Suppl. 11, 906.

CURRIERI, P. W. & LUTERMAN, A.(1978) Nutritional Support of the Burned Patient. *Surg. Clin. N. Am.,* **58**, 1151.

DAVIDSON, S., PASSMORE, R.*et al.* (1979) *Human Nutrition and Dietetics.* 7th edn. Churchill Livingstone, Edinburgh.

DAVIES, J. W. L. & FELL, G. S.(1974) Tissue Catabolism in Patients with Burns. *Clin. Chim. Acta,* **51**, 83.

HILDRETH, M. & CARVAJAH, H. F.(1982) Caloric Requirements in Burned Children. *J. Burn Care Rehab.,* **3**, 78.

HILL, G. L.(1981) *Nutrition and the Surgical Patient.* Churchill Livingstone, London.

KINNEY, J. M.(1979) Protein Metabolism in Burned Patients. *J. Trauma,* **19**, Suppl. 11, 900.

SAFFLE, J. R., MEDINA, E.*et al.* (1985) Indirect Calorimetry in the Burned Patient. *J. Trauma,* **25**, 32.

SEROG, P., BAIGHTS, F.*et al.* (1983) Energy and Nitrogen Balances in 24 Burned Patients. *Burns,* **9**, 422.

SUTHERLAND, A. B.(1976) Nitrogen Balance and Nutritional Requirement in the Burned Patient. *Burns,* **2**, 238.

SUTHERLAND, A. B. & BATCHELOR, A. D. R.(1966) Nitrogen Balance in Burned Children. *Research in Burns: Trans. 2nd Int. Congr. on Burns.* Churchill Livingstone, Edinburgh.

TURNER, W. W., IRETON, C. S.*et al.* (1985) Energy Expenditures in Burned Patients. *J. Trauma,* **25**, 11.

20

Scars and Contractures

Burns which are dermal or full-thickness produce scarring. Grafts appear within the first few months to be free of scar, but later may pucker and contract, before eventually maturing and flattening.

The aim of scar management is firstly its prevention or minimizing, and secondly, release of established contracture.

Prevention and Minimizing Scars and Scar Contracture

Grafting

Deep dermal burns, though they may heal spontaneously after a few weeks, tend to produce an unsatisfactory amount of scarring. Provided the condition of the patient permits, and the extent of the surface to be grafted is not extensive, it is preferable to graft these deep dermal burns to produce a better quality scar than would occur with spontaneous healing. This is especially indicated if the burn is over a joint where contracture may be anticipated.

Positioning

Correct positioning of the anatomical part during the healing phase may prevent contracture occurring.

Limbs

Limbs are elevated above the level of the shoulder or groin to facilitate lymphatic and venous return.

Hands

Frequent regular active and passive movements of the wrists, metacarpophalangeal and interphalangeal joints through a full range are insisted upon. The hands are placed in polythene bags (plastic refrigerator–freezer bags are sterile), with a lightly applied crepe bandage to hold it in place around the forearm (Fig. 10.2 p.71).

Alternatively the hand is dressed with Bactigras tulle, gauze, cotton wool and bandaged. The position of bandaging is important and is often only maintained by incorporating a plaster of Paris or Aquaplast splint into the bandage:

The thumb is abducted fully, with a foam pad in the first web space.

The wrist is extended to 20°

The metacarpophalangeal joints are flexed to 90°

The interphalangeal joints are straight (Fig. 20.1).

Where skin loss on the dorsum of the interphalangeal joints is deep or full thickness, passive or active attempts at flexion may expose or rupture the extensor digitorum tendon, resulting in boutonnière deformity. In such cases early skin grafting is preferable to delay and attempts at stretching.

In general, joints are splinted in extension (with the exception of the metacarpophalangeal joints of the hand) since flexion contracture is more difficult to overcome than extension.

The elbow

During burn healing, the elbow is splinted 10° short of straight, but is put through a full range of motion several times on at least three occasions a day.

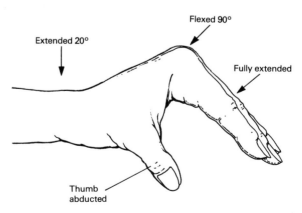

Fig. 20.1 Position of wrist, thumb and fingers immobilized in a bandage

The shoulder

For axillary and upper arm burns, the patient is nursed with the shoulder abducted, either by copious dressing paddings in the axilla or, if the burn is exposed, by supporting the abducted arms on several pillows or foam bricks.

The neck

For burns of the neck the pillows are placed beneath the scapulae, not behind the head. The neck is extended.

If the burn is dressed, a bulky foam collar may be incorporated over the dressings to elevate the chin.

Popliteal fossa

For burns in the popliteal fossa, bulky dressings or pillows behind the knee are avoided, so that the knee is fully extended. If the patient is sitting in a chair, flexion of the knees is prevented by elevating the legs onto a footstool.

Ankle

Flexion of the ankle and foot–drop is controlled by placing right-angled plastic splints beneath the feet, adequately padded over the contact with the heel. Hexcelite or Aquaplast are convenient thermoplastic materials available from the occupational or physio-therapy department from which these splints may be moulded. Alternatively, a footboard or large blocks of polythene bricks may be used against the soles of the feet. To provide movement of the ankles, a sling under the sole, when pulled upon by the patient's hands, passively extends them.

When the patient is lying prone, the feet hang over the bottom of the mattress.

Ambulation

Early and repeated ambulation is carried out.

Joint Movement

Each joint is put through its full range of movement several times a day.

Hypertrophic Scarring

Burns scars may become raised, itchy and red within one or two months of healing (Fig. 20.2). Indeed the itchiness may become the most uncomfortable part of the healing process. Not only are these scars unsightly, especially when on the face, but they contribute to

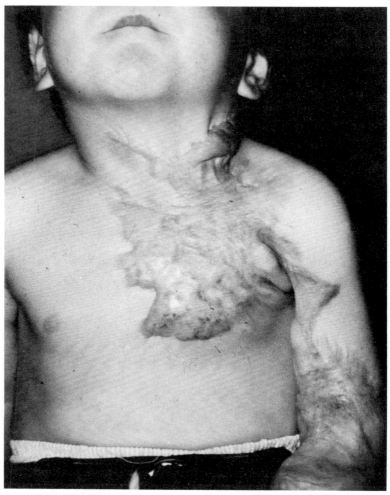

Fig. 20.2   Hypertrophic scar

joint contracture and limitation of range of joint movement. Areas of the body particularly likely to develop hypertrophic scars are the pre-sternal and sub-mandibular regions.

Prevention

1 Early release of tension. Deep burns over flexion creases of joints, though eventually healing spontaneously, do so under tension. There is some evidence that tension in a scar encourages hypertrophy, so that early grafting of such burns may mitigate this.
2 Pressure on maturing scar tissue appears to reduce the incidence of hypertrophic change. Pressure is most readily maintained by elasticated garments, Tubegrip sleeves or made-to-measure Jobst★ or Panmed garments (Fig. 20.3).

Such pressure has to be maintained 24 hours per day for 6 to 12 months. The earlier that pressure treatment is started the more effective it appears to be, in practice as soon as the wound is healed and stable.

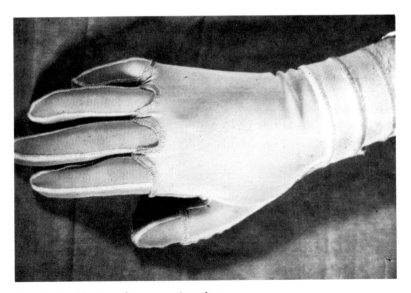

Fig. 20.3   Elasticated compression glove

★ Jobst Centre, 17 Wigmore Street, London, W.1. Tel: 01-629-6943; Panmed Ltd. Eddison Road, Churchfields, Salisbury, Wiltshire. Tel: 0722-21422

Treatment of Established Hypertrophic Scar

1 Release of tension. Where contractures are occurring, their release by the insertion of skin grafts (or occasionally by rearranging the tissues locally by Z-plasty) may result in recession of the hypertrophy.
2 Injection of triamcinolone acetonide (1–2 ml of 25 mg/ml) into the hypertrophic scar, on two or three occasions at approximately one-monthly intervals. Care should be taken that the steroid does not enter the sub-scar fat where it would cause tissue lysis.
3 Massaging a bland cream into the scar may help to lubricate and soften the hypertrophy, and gives the patient some reassurance. Aqueous cream BP or Hydrous Ointment BP are usually satisfactory. Ointments and applications containing steroid have been popular but there is no evidence of their effectiveness, and they may permit development of local infection if there is a break in the epidermis.
4 Itching may be alleviated with calamine compound 10% BP or calamine lotion 15% BP.
5 Reassurance is given that the natural history of hypertrophic scars is ultimately one of flattening and softening, with loss of redness and itching (though this may take up to 2 or 3 years in refractory cases).

Keloids

It is important to make the distinction between keloids and hypertrophic scars (Table 20.1), because their behaviour is different.

Table 20.1   Characteristics of keloids and hypertrophic scars.

	Hypertrophic scar	*Keloid*
Incidence		High in Negro skins
Extent	Confined to site of injury	Extends into surrounding uninjured skin
Result	Tends to become flat after a few years	Persists and enlarges
Recurrence	Some tendency to recur after excision	High tendency to recur after excision

Whereas treatment for a hypertrophic scar is expectant towards eventual spontaneous improvement, such a favourable outcome is lacking with keloid. When the keloid is incapacitating or unacceptable in appearance, it may be excised within its margins (to avoid surgical damage to skin outside the area of scarring) and skin grafted. The incidence of recurrence is high.

Treatment of Established Contracture

If scar contractures are not released, secondary contracture occurs in joint capsules making correction difficult if not impossible. It is judicious therefore not to delay contracture release, though of course prevention is preferable.

Minor degrees of contracture may be released by local rearrangement of adjacent skin, by Z-plasties. The value of this method is very limited in burns because it rarely provides sufficient extensible tissue to provide a satisfactory release.

Most established contractures require incision into scar band, extending the incision until the band is fully released and the joint moveable through its full range. The resultant defect is closed with a medium partial-thickness skin graft, and the joint splinted in extension until the graft has taken and for a few days afterwards.

Joints in children may be splinted for several weeks without the danger of joint stiffness, but adults' joints will not normally tolerate immobilization for more than a week or two. For the more refractory contractures, this release regimen may be necessary several times over two or three years.

Scar contractures around the eyes produce ectropion and on the fingers flexion or extension joint deformities. Such deformities are best treated by incision to release the contracture, and closure of the defect with full-thickness skin grafts (from the groin or behind the ears). These full-thickness grafts do not shrink as partial thickness grafts do.

Occasionally, when bone, joint or cartilage is exposed by contracture release, or when skin grafting has been unsatisfactory, a flap of skin and fat may be used to close the defect resulting after incision and release of the contracture.

Long-standing Scars

Repeated ulceration of an unstable burn scar, or of a scar subject to recurrent trauma may, after many years, lead to malignant change (Marjolin's ulcer), usually basal or squamous cell carcinoma.

Fibrosarcoma has been described in long-standing burn scars.

Such scars therefore require release, excision, regrafting or flap cover to the defect, long before malignant change supervenes.

References

EDSTROM, L.E., ROBSON, M.C. & HEADLEY, B.J. (1978) Exercise Techniques in the Burn Patient. *Burns,* **4**, 113.

FELLER, I. & GRABB, W.C. (1979) *Reconstruction and Rehabilitation of the Burned Patient.* National Institute for Burn Patients, Ann Arbour, Michigan 48104.

HEAD, M.D. & HELM, P.A. (1978) Sustained Stretching in Burn Contractures. *Burns,* **4**, 136.

JACKSON, D.M. (1980) Destructive Burns : some Orthopaedic Complications. *Burns,* **7**, 105.

KEMBLE, J.V.H. (1976) Scarring Electromicroscopy of the Hypertrophic Scar. *Postgrad. Med. J.,* **52**, 219.

KIRSCHER, C.W. & SHETLAR, M.R. (1979) Microvasculature in Hypertrophic Scars and the Effects of Pressure. *J. Trauma,* **19**, 757.

KLOT, J. & POCHON, J.P. (1982) Compression Suits for Burns in Children. *Burns,* **8**, 180.

LARSON, D.L., ABSTON, S., EVANS, E.B. & LINARES, H.A.(1971) Techniques for Decreasing Scar Formation in the Burned Patient. *J. Trauma,* **11**, 801.

LARSON, D.L., BAUR, P., LINARES, H.A., WILLIS, B., ABSTON, S. & LEWIS, S.R. (1974) Mechanisms of Hypertrophic Scar and Contracture Formation in Burns. *Burns,* **1**, 119.

LEUNG, P.C. & NG, M. (1980) Pressure Treatment for Hypertrophic Scars. *Burns,* **6**, 244.

LINARES, H.A. & LARSON, D.L. (1976) Elastic Tissue and Hypertrophic Scars. *Burns,* **3**, 4.

NICOSIA, J., STEIN, E.D. & STEIN, J.M. (1980) Physiotherapy for Burns Patients under Anaesthesia. *Burns,* **6**, 202.

SHAKESPEARE, P.G. & RENTERGHEM, L. VAN. (1985) Surface Structure of Collagen in Hypertrophic Scars. *Burns,* **11**, 175.

STERN, P.J., NEALE, H.W. *et al.* (1985) Management of Burned Thumb Contractures in Children. *Burns,* **11**, 168.

TROTT, J.A. & HOBBY, J.A.E. (1978) Burns of the Female Breast. *Burns,* **4**, 267.

WAGNER, M.M. (1981) *Care of the Burn Injured Patient.* Croom Helm, London.

21

Burns of Special Sites

Hands

Since persistent oedematous fluid organizes to collagen, it is imperative to minimize scarring within the hand by promoting lymphatic and venous drainage. The burned hand should be elevated above the level of the shoulder at all times.

Drainage can also be promoted by frequent and regular muscular movement of the hand and forearm. For this reason it is convenient to place the hand in a clear polythene bag (large enterostomy bags or deep freeze food container bags are satisfactory (Fig. 10.2)), and bandage it around the forearm with a lightly applied conforming bandage. The patient and physiotherapist can then see that the full range of finger movement is achieved.

Any exudate will collect in the bag which can be changed as frequently as necessary. If required a small amount of silver sulphadiazine may be incorporated into the bag.

Full-thickness burns of the hands should be excised and grafted in the theatre within 4 or 5 days of injury, to enable early movement of the hand to be started. The grafts are usually best sutured into place for stability, and movement of the fingers begun as soon as the graft is reasonably secure, under physiotherapy supervision. While the grafts are stabilizing the hand is bandaged with the interphalangeal joints fully extended, the finger metacarpophalangeal joints flexed to 90° and the thumb abducted (Fig. 20.1).

Exposure by burn injury of distal interphalangeal joints of the fingers is usually best treated by amputation just proximal to the joint. Exposure of extensor tendons on the back of hand does not necessitate their removal as small areas can often be bridged by a graft.

Splintage of the hand while the patient is asleep at night helps to prevent contracture into non-functional postures. A resting or night splint should ensure the fingers are extended fully at the interphalangeal joints, flexed to 90° at the finger metacarpophalangeal joints, and the thumb fully abducted. (See splintage p.200).

175

Ears

Exposure treatment is the most satisfactory, the ear being kept clean with saline, gently debrided and covered with silver sulphadiazine cream, applied at least daily. Even exposed cartilage will often granulate and allow epithelialization. Excision of cartilage often leads to a worse deformity than leaving it in place.

Eyelids

Full-thickness eyelid burns need to be treated urgently since exposure of the cornea leads to ulceration and blindness. Until the patient is fit for operation, the eyes are kept clean with saline and chloramphenicol ointment is instilled 2 hourly. Eye pads are best avoided since they may scratch the cornea. Contact lenses are easily overlooked. They must be specifically enquired about and removed. (See also page 180).

Grafting with thick split skin is undertaken when slough has separated and some granulations have formed. It is essential to ensure that the cornea is never allowed to dry. The grafting will probably need to be repeated on several occasions as the grafts contract, and over-correction is advisable.

Partial-thickness burns cause gross eyelid and conjunctival swelling soon making examination of the eyes impossible. Ophthalmological examination must take place before oedema closes the lids. Fluorescein drops will make corneal damage visible. Fluid trapped behind the swollen lids is released, at least hourly, by gently opening a gap between them; a Desmarre retractor is useful for this. The eye and lids are cleaned with saline and kept covered with chloramphenicol ointment. Attempts to obtain lid adhesion by tarsorraphy usually fails because of the friability of the tissues and the tension caused by the oedema.

Mouth

Mouth burns most commonly occur as a result of children sucking live electrical wires. There is considerable anguish both in the child and the parent.

Primary excision is inadvisable since in the early days uninjured tissue may be needlessly removed. After about 10 days, necrotic tissue is apparent and can be debrided. Reconstruction is by mucosal advancement and local flaps.

Face

With the exception of burns due to flash, facial burning from flame will arouse suspicion of inhalation injury. The lax tissue allows enormous degrees of oedema, not only tightly closing the eyelids, but swelling the lips and tongue. Explanation to patient and relatives about the temporary distortion of the face for 6–8 days allays subsequent concern.

After cleaning with saline, beard and head hair is clipped to allow better toilet. The patient is nursed well propped up on pillows to encourage drainage. A nasogastric tube is inserted before the nasal mucosa swells blocking the airway.

Diagnosis of the depth of burning on the face is difficult and early excision is contraindicated. It is often surprising how much facial skin regenerates. The face is cleaned regularly with saline and lightly covered with an antiseptic such as silver sulphadiazine. Crusting and drying should not be permitted.

For deep partial-thickness burns, some of the fluid loss and pain may be reduced by applying autograft, or (if not available or required for full-thickness burned areas) homograft skin.

Before full thickness burns begin to granulate, sheets of autograft are applied in facial units (i.e. complete sheet for the cheek, for the nose, for the forehead, for the upper lip and for the chin). The grafts are immobilized onto the face by means of sutures using the quilting technique to secure the centre as well as the edges of the grafts (like an eiderdown quilt).

Neck

Correct positioning of the neck (see p. 169) reduces the amount of many neck contractures. To release a tight neck contracture (Fig. 21.1), a transverse curved incision is made at the angle of neck and submental region over the hyoid. Grafts are sutured, padded and held in place with a plastozote collar (page 191).

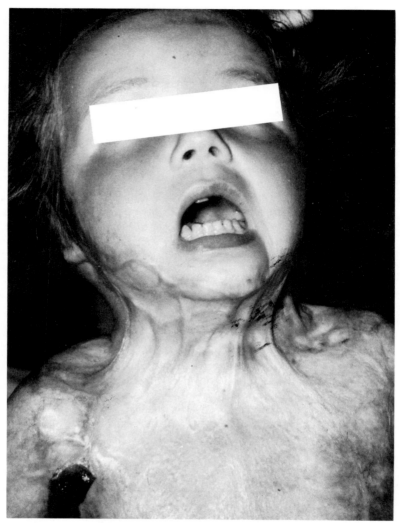

Fig. 21.1   Neck contracture

References

ALEXANDER, J.W., MACMILLAN, B.G. & MARTEL, L. (1982) Correction of Postburn Syndactily. *Plastic Recon. Surg.,* **70**, 345.
DOWLING, J.A., FOLEY, F.D. & MONCRIEF, J.A. (1968) Chondritis in the Burned Ear. *Plastic Recon. Surg.,* **42**, 115.

FRANK, D.H., WACHTEL, T. & FRANK, H.A. (1983) Treatment and Reconstruction of Eyelid Burns. *J. Trauma*, **23**, 874.

FRAUDSEN, P.A., NIELSEN, H.O. & SOMMER, J. (1977) Second Degree Burns of the Hand. *Burns*, **4**, 20.

GOEL, T.K., LAW, E.J., LAW, E.J. & MACMILLAN, B.G. (1982) Management of the Acutely Burned Ear. *Burns*, **9**, 218.

GOODWIN, C.W., MAGUIRE, M.S., MCMANUS, W.F. & PRUITT, B.A. (1983) Study of Burn Wound Excision of the Hands. *J. Trauma*, **23**, 510.

HARNAR, T., ENGRAV, L. *et al.* (1985) Skeletal Immobilisation of Burned Hands. *J. Trauma*, **25**, 299.

JACKSON, D.M. & HALL, M.J.R. (1980) Preservation of Sight after Complete Destruction of the Eyelids. *Burns*, **7**, 221.

KRIZEK, T.J., FLAGG, S.V., WOLFORT, F.G. & JABALEY, M.E. (1973) Delayed Primary Excision and Skin Grafting of the Burned Hand. *Plastic Recon. Surg.*, **51**, 524.

LEUNG, P.C. & CHOW, Y.Y.N. (1981) Treatment of Burned Hands. *Burns*, **8**, 338.

MORGAN, R.F. & NICHTER, L.S. (1985) Management of Head and Neck Burns. *J. Burn Care Rehab.*, **6**, 20.

NIELSEN, A.B. & SOMMER, J. (1982) Surgical Treatment of the Deeply Burned Hand. *Burns*, **9**, 214.

SALISBURY, R.E. & WRIGHT, P. (1982) Early Excision of Dorsal Hand Burns. *Plastic Recon. Surg.*, **69**, 670.

SKOOG, T. (1963) The Surgical Treatment of Burns. *Acta Chir. Scand. Suppl.*, 305.

SOEDA, S. & NAKAYAMA, Y. (1980) Nasal Deformities due to Burns. *Burns*, **6**, 266.

STERN, P.J., NEAL, H.W. *et al.* (1985) Management of Burn Thumb Contractures in Children. *Burns*, **11**, 168.

SYKES, P.J. & BAILEY, B.N. (1976) Treatment of Hand Burns with Occlusive Bags. *Burns*, **2**, 162.

WACHTEL, T.L. & FRANK, D.H. (1984) *Burns of the Head and Neck*. W.B. Saunders, Philadelphia.

22

Late Surgery for Burns

The Eyelids

Burns ectropion requires corrective surgery, often on several occasions, before conjunctivitis and keratitis supervene. The wearing of occlusive spectacles or goggles, and use of eye ointments are only short-lasting and temporary expedients.

Under general anaesthesia (or local anaesthesia if necessary), a transverse incision is made about 2 mm above or below the eyelid margin, until the lid can be inturned to lie against the globe in its proper position. An exact pattern of the resulting defect is taken in aluminium foil (the suture aluminium wrapper is convenient). The pattern is transferred to the angle between the scalp and medial aspect of the ear, or above the clavicle; the shape and size of the pattern is marked out on the skin with Bonney's blue, and the appropriate piece of full-thickness skin excised. Care is taken not to crush the tissue, holding it only with skin hooks.

All subdermal fat is carefully removed from the graft with iris scissors. The full-thickness graft is laid into the eyelid defect, having first ensured that the bed is free from bleeding.

Using 5/0 nylon or silk, the graft is sutured into the defect, skin-edge to graft-edge. One end of each suture is left 5 cm (2 in) long.

The graft is now covered with one layer of vaseline tulle gras, exactly the same size and shape as the graft. A bolus of sterilized foam or proflavine wool is laid onto the tulle gras, and the long ends of the sutures tied to each other over the bolus to hold it in place (Fig. 22.1).

Any blood in the conjunctival sac is washed out with saline and chloramphenicol ointment is instilled into the eye.

The bolus and sutures may be removed after 5 days by which time the graft should have 'taken' on the bed.

Preparation of Proflavine Wool

Flavine emulsion is heated to lukewarm, and good quality cotton wool is thoroughly mixed into it. The wool is then wrung out to

180

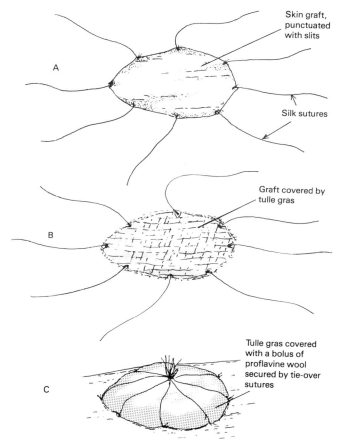

A — Skin graft, punctuated with slits

Silk sutures

B — Graft covered by tulle gras

C — Tulle gras covered with a bolus of proflavine wool secured by tie-over sutures

Fig. 22.1 The 'tie-over' dressing. A, skin graft sutured on to burn site; B, graft covered with tulle gras; C, tulle gras covered with a bolus of proflavine wool or foam and secured by tying the long ends of the sutures together at the centre

remove excess emulsion: the wool should now feel dry. It is placed in a warm cupboard to remove the remaining moisture. After autoclaving, it is ready for use.

Eyebrows

Where eyebrow hair has been destroyed, an eyebrow pencil may be sufficient simulation (particularly for women). However, the eyebrow may be reconstructed by grafting a hair-bearing strip of skin into the eyebrow region.

A strip of occipital scalp hair-bearing skin is satisfactory. When removing the graft from the occiput, the scalpel is inclined at the angle at which the hairs emerge from the skin, so as to ensure that the follicles are not incised. Since the graft is often being placed into somewhat avascular burned tissue, the width of the graft should not exceed about 4 mm.

The direction of the hairs should be orientated so that their direction of lie is medial to lateral.

The strip is immobilized with fine sutures around its circumference and tied over a bolus in the same way as for a full-thickness graft to the eyelid.

A superficial temporal artery pedicled hair-bearing flap from the temporal scalp instead of a free occipital graft has been used, but gives rather a thick exuberant eyebrow.

Mouth

Microstoma caused by scar contractures around the mouth may have a serious detrimental effect on patient's nutrition. It should be corrected by full-thickness incisions at each side of the mouth opening, as far as a line dropped vertically from the pupil of the eye (looking straight ahead).

Oral mucosa is mobilized by undermining for 1–2 cm, and everted onto the lip skin to which it is sutured. The new commissure of the mouth is 'fish-tailed'.

Nose

Where scarring is unacceptable after all hypertrophic change has subsided, the entire surface of the nose may be grafted using a single partial-thickness sheet. The scar is firstly deeply dermabraded using a rotating carborundum cylinder on a dental drill. Bleeding is controlled, and the sheet graft applied, suturing it around its edges at the glabella, angle of nose with cheek and inside the margin of the nares to the nasal mucosa.

Care must be taken not to expose nasal cartilage when dermabrading, since grafts will then fail.

When the nose has been destroyed, flap reconstruction is required. Since the forehead has often also been burned, this is not available, and more distant sites such as the top of the scalp (if the patient is bald) or the flexor aspect of the upper arm tax and ingenuity of the plastic surgeon and the stamina of the patient.

Prosthetic reconstruction, with a skin-toned acrylic prosthesis mounted on a spectacle frame or applied with glue is often a very satisfactory compromise, particularly for the more elderly. Such prostheses are often a work of art by maxillo-facial technicians.

The Neck

Much can be done to prevent neck contracture, by correct positioning of the head in extension during the healing phase, and the prolonged wearing of a plastozote cervical collar.

Severe flexion contracture may prevent anaesthesia by endotracheal intubation. In such cases, the scar may have to be released under local anaesthesia, intubation and general anaesthesia commenced and then the release and reconstruction completed.

Relieving incisions should be transverse and extend well round to the side of the neck. Small bands may be released by Z-plasty, though these are the minority. Usually one, or two large sheets of thick partial-thickness skin graft are required. They are sewn into the defect, held in place with a bolus of foam or proflavine wool tied in as for eyelid grafts, and immobilized in a cervical collar.

A collar should be worn for at least 6 months day and night to prevent re-contracture.

Axilla, Antecubital Fossa, Popliteal Fossa

Established contractures (Fig. 22.2) are usually inadequately released by Z-plasty, and require thick partial-thickness skin grafts to the released skin defect. The grafts are kept in contact with the bed with a conforming foam or proflavine wool bolus.

Splints of plaster of Paris, or better, since they are lighter, of Hexcelite, are applied on the operating table, so that no movement occurs at the joint to shear the grafts. Splintage should be maintained for several weeks until the patient can put the joint through a full range of movement.

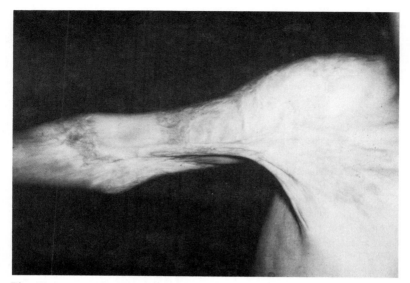

Fig. 22.2   Axillary contracture

Dorsum of Foot and Toes

Release of the extension contracture often exposes the toe extensor tendons. Grafts will take satisfactorily provided the paratenon is intact, but tenotomy may be necessary to allow the toe to drop into its proper position.

The Hand

Dorsal burns produce hyperextension of the metacarpophalangeal joints and boutonnière deformity of the fingers (due to burning of the central slip of the extensor tendon). Subluxation of the joints accompanies severe contracture, and capsular contracture occurs in adults after a few weeks of immobilization of the metacarpo-phalangeal joint in extension.

The hyperextension deformity is relieved by a transverse incision across the distal part of the back of the hand. Extensor tendon paratenon should be carefully preserved, and a thick partial-thickness skin graft sutured into the defect, held in place with a bolus of foam or proflavine wool.

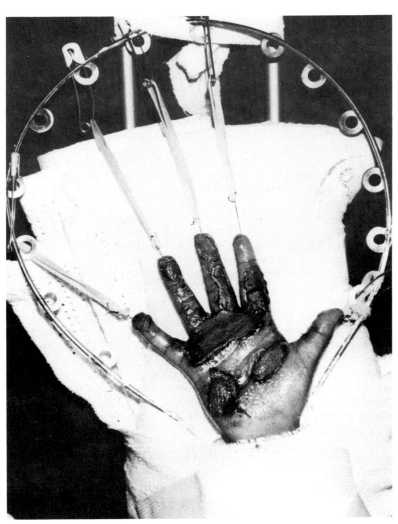

Fig. 22.3 Banjo splint (See p.207)

The hand and fingers are immobilized in a plaster of Paris slab or Hexcelite splint on the volar aspect from forearm to finger tips with the metacarpophalangeal joints flexed to 90° and interphalangeal joints straight (Fig. 20.1) until the graft is stable (usually about 7 days).

In severe cases of joint capsule contracture, capsulotomy may be necessary. The joint is immobilized by a trans-articular Kirschner wire for 3 weeks, with the joint in as much flexion as can be gained.

The boutonnière deformity may be corrected by releasing the two lateral slips of the extensor tendon and plicating them onto the dorsum of the proximal interphalangeal joint with Dexon. The joint is immobilized with a trans-articular Kirschner wire for 3 weeks, or by external splintage.

Arthrodesis of the proximal interphalangeal joint in 45° of flexion with a polypropylene (Harrison) peg or crossed Kirschner wires is often the only reasonable solution to destruction of the central extensor slip.

When the hyperextension of the terminal interphalangeal joint is marked, tenotomy of the extensor tendon lateral slips just proximal to the distal interphalangeal joint will allow the terminal phalanx to drop to the neutral position.

Palmar burns, often from grasping electric fire filaments, occur mostly in children. The interdigital spaces are often webbed (burns syndactily). These may be released by double Z-plasty, using thick partial-thickness or full-thickness skin grafts to the residual defects. To facilitate cleaning and inspection of the grafts, the fingers are partially immobilized on a 'banjo splint' with elastic bands attached to the finger nails (Fig. 22.3).

Since these hands are so small, they can often only be satisfactorily splinted by complete enveloping splints. The oyster splint, made in two (dorsal and palmar) halves, moulded closely to the hand, is useful. If the mould has to be made on a recently grafted hand, the graft may be protected by covering the hand in a polythene bag (page 205).

References

Much of the later reconstructive procedures for burns involve specialist surgery. Only general references are therefore given here.

ARTZ, C. P., MONCRIEF, J. A. & PRUITT, B. A.(1979) *Burns – a Team Approach.* W. B. Saunders, Philadelphia.

CASON, J. S.(1981) *Treatment of Burns.* Chapman and Hall, London.

CONVERSE, J. M.(1977) *Reconstructive Plastic Surgery; Principles and Procedures in Correction, Reconstruction and Transplantation.* W. B. Saunders, Philadelphia.

FELLER, I. & GRABB, W. C.(1979) *Reconstruction and Rehabilitation of the Burned Patient*. National Institute for Burn Patients, Ann Arbour, Michigan 48104.

GRABB, W. C. & SMITH, J. W.(1979) *Plastic Surgery*. Little, Brown, Boston.

MCDOUGALL, W. S., SLADE, C. L. & PRUITT, B. A.(1978) *Manual of Burns*. Springer, New York.

WACHTEL, T. L. & FRANK, D. H.(1984) *Burns of the Head and Neck*. W. B. Saunders, Philadelphia.

WATSON, J. & MCCORMACK, R.(1979) *Operative Surgery – Fundamental International Techniques*. Butterworth, London.

23

Practical Aspects of Splintage

The principles of splinting in treatment of the burn patient are based on those which apply to splinting any patient. It is emphasized that particular care and thought must be given to the comfort of the patient, to good joint position and to the avoidance of pressure. The aim of these notes is to help those occupational therapists who have limited experience of splinting the burn patient.

Indications for Splinting

The indications for splintage for the burn patient include:
1 The maintenance of good joint position to prevent the formation of disabling contractures as healing takes place. With correct positioning of the patient, splinting may be avoided or kept to a minimum; however, the very ill patient may be unable to co-operate in positioning, or the area burned may need a more rigid support than can be achieved with pillows or foam blocks.
2 The prevention of contracture after grafting.
3 After grafting, the immobilization of an area until the graft has become stable.
4 The stretching of contracted skin.
5 To help to overcome oedema.
6 The protection of an exposed tendon.
In some instances, static splinting may be sufficient and in others, dynamic splinting is preferred. The indications for static or dynamic splinting are as follows:

Dynamic Splinting

1 When an element of gradual stretch is required e.g. contracted skin.
2 When it is necessary to maintain joint movement while at the same time preventing contractures forming.

Static Splinting

1 When it is necessary to maintain a joint position while healing takes place.
2 For postgrafting immobilization.
3 When stretch is required, but it is not possible to make a dynamic splint for technical reasons, a static splint is used with serial alteration.
4 The protection of exposed tendons.

Materials and Equipment

When the general condition of the patient confines him to the ward, splints are made at the patient's bedside. This necessitates making splints with limited equipment and facilities. It is therefore necessary to use designs which are simple. Paper patterns may be impractical in many situations and measurements with a tape measure are likely to be more feasible.

Materials Used

For hands, wrists and necks **Sansplint XR** is the chosen material as it has a stretch factor which makes it conform easily in those areas where an exact fit is necessary. Other, similar, thermoplastic materials such as **Orthoplast,Orfit, Aquaplast** or **Sansplint** are also suitable.

For all other splints **Hexcelite** is preferred as it is easily handled for the larger splints, has better ventilation properties, and can be readily reinforced by the addition of extra layers of material. It requires padding to protect the skin if the patient does not have dressings.

To use these materials the suppliers' instructions are followed.

Padding Materials

High density adhesive foams are used for padding hand splints. These are available in various thicknesses and have different properties specified by the suppliers. Alternatively, adhesive orthopaedic felt is used. Gamgee is used to line splints made from Hexcelite or, for a very light lining, stockinette is used.

Finger Slings

Leatherette with one side bonded to stockinette is used for finger slings or elbow pads.

Equipment

A multicooker electric pan for heating water is used for moulding thermosplastic materials in the ward or operating theatre. In the later stages of treatment, when the patient can come to the therapy department, hydrocolators of many types are suitable. Other tools include scissors and shears of personal choice, six-way leather punch, tape measure.

Fastenings

In the recently burned patient it is best to use bandages to secure splints in order to spread pressure evenly over the limb and to avoid putting a constrictive band on affected skin. This is particularly important when oedema is present. At later stages, when healing has taken place and when the patient is capable of looking after his own splint, Velcro straps are more convenient and acceptable. These are very quick and easy to fit and are used in conjuction with small pieces of self-adhesive Velcro which are fixed to the splint at appropriate positions.

Splinting with Exercise

Splints form part of a planned programme of wear, alternating with exercise, with exercise periods gradually predominating. Many patients can quickly adopt a timetable of wearing their splints at night only, while also wearing pressure garments (Jobst or Panmed). These garments considerably reduce the length of time splints need to be worn. Progress needs to be carefully monitored.

Aftercare

It is very important that splints are checked by the therapist at frequent intervals. When made to fit over dressings, checks should be done whenever the dressing is changed. Inevitably there is some variation in bulk or extent of dressings and small alterations may need to be done frequently to ensure a good fit.

The therapist instructs nurses caring for the patient on the correct application of the splint, including positioning and bandaging. The nurse is responsible for understanding and implementing these instructions.

As in all splint procedures, the patient is given clear information on the reason for the splint and how it will work to achieve the objectives. Even when very ill and apparently unresponsive to events around him, the patient is told simply but clearly that a splint is being made to keep his leg/arm in the correct position. When he goes home the patient is given written instructions including:

1 When the splint should be worn and when taken off for exercise.
2 How to care for the splint.
3 A phone number to ring and name of the therapist in case of any problems which might arise with the splint.
4 The date and place for follow-up appointments for splint checks.

Specific Areas Which May Require Splinting

Neck

It is important to maintain the right angle of the neck with the jaw. Extremely disfiguring and disabling contractures occur when this angle is lost and the chin becomes flexed towards the chest. There are several methods of controlling these contractures:

1 For a partial thickness burn A **soft collar** such as those used in the treatment of neck pain is sufficient. For children, a soft collar can be made using orthopaedic felt, in length 2.5 cm (1 in) less than the circumference of the child's neck and width to the full height of the neck. This is then inserted into a length of Tubigrip (Seton Ltd) of sufficient length to use the end to tie the collar at the back of the neck.
2 A **pneumatic collar** (Fig 23.1) gives slightly more control than the soft collar.
3 A **thermoplastic collar** (Fig. 23.2) is necessary for a full-thickness burn or where a soft or blow-up collar fails to control contracture. Sansplint XR is the best material to use, as the ability to stretch is necessary for a successful fit.

Construction of neck collaɪ

An ellipse is drawn as shown in Fig. 23.3 and the shape is cut out from Sansplint XR. Soften as instructed.

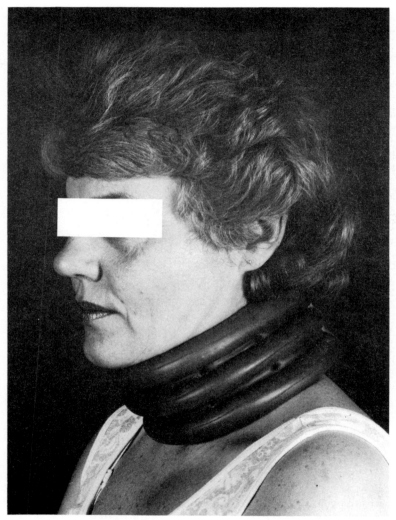

Fig. 23.1   Rubber neck collar

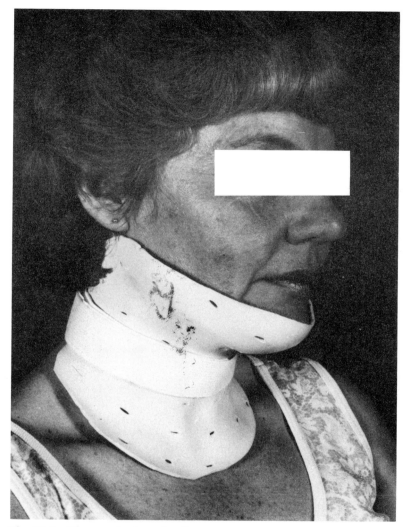

Fig. 23.2 Thermoplastic neck collar

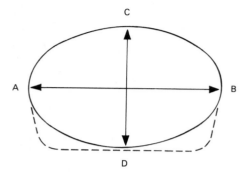

Fig. 23.3   Neck collar pattern

Measurement A → B = measurement around neck from ear to ear.
Measurement C → D = measurement from 1 cm (½ in) above chin
to 2.5 cm (1 in) below sternoclavicular joint.

Moulding

Two people are needed for this. Person 1, standing in front of the
patient, holds point C of the softened material in position on the
patient's chin and smooths the material onto the neck to the
conformity required.

Meanwhile, person 2, standing behind the patient gently pulls at
points A and B to stretch the material slightly round the neck. If the
burn extends to the side of the neck, the splint is cut to a squarer
shape at the lower edge, as shown by the dotted line on Fig. 23.3.
This extends the splint onto the shoulder and prevents lateral neck
contracture.

The lower edge is flared away from the skin to prevent pressure.
This edge may need padding.

A light dressing is put between the patient's neck and the splint. It
is also necessary to remove the splint frequently to wash and dry it,
as maceration can occur if the skin is allowed to become wet.

Axilla

A burn occurring under or at the sides of the upper arm or on the
chest wall around and in the axilla, needs an 'aeroplane' splint to
prevent the formation of contracture that would limit abduction of
the arm at the shoulder.

Similarly if a release of an old burn contracture or a graft has been performed, this type of splint will be needed. The splint is made to abduct the shoulder up to 90° (see Fig. 23.4).

Construction

These splints are made from Hexcelite and although several variations may be made for the arm support, the basic principles of construction remain the same. The splint is made in three parts (Fig. 23.5).

1 A 15 cm (6 in) width of Hexcelite, one-third the length of patients' waist circumference, is heated and folded over 3.5 cm (1.5 in) webbing, cut to waist measurement, plus 7 cm (3 in) extra for fastening overlap. While soft, this is moulded to the side of the waist. The inside of this should be well padded.

2 A spar is made from a 20 cm (8 in) width of Hexcelite rolled over on itself. This joins the waistband to the arm support. For an adult this needs further reinforcing with strips of Hexcelite.

3 The arm support is made from double-thickness Hexcelite and moulded to fit the lower half of the upper arm, allowing sufficient space for padding. Particular care should be taken on padding the distal end if supporting only the upper arm. If the burn extends over the elbow, the arm support may be made to support the

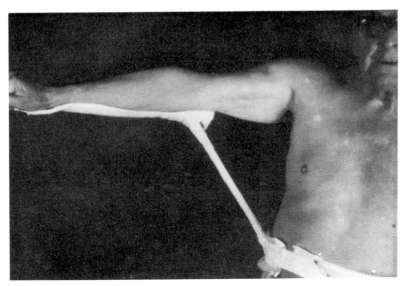

Fig. 23.4   Aeroplane arm splint

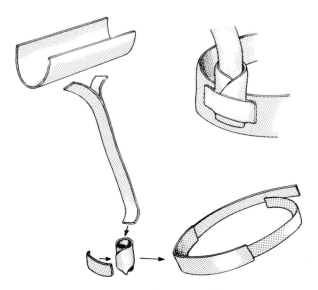

Fig. 23.5 Pattern for aeroplane arm splint

whole arm. It should then reach to the palmar crease of the hand, in order to support the wrist. The three parts are fused together in the positions shown using small pieces of softened Hexcelite.

Most patients prefer the upper arm support to the whole arm splint as it gives more freedom of movement to the hand. Support may be given to the forearm with pillows if needed.

Fastening

The arm is bandaged to the upper arm support. The waistband webbing is overlapped and secured with large safety pins.

Elbow

The aim of splinting here is to combat flexion contracture resulting from a burn on the flexor aspect of the elbow.

Static splinting may be achieved by making a half cylinder of Hexcelite to fit over the flexor aspect. This is possible if the burn area is dressed and padded.

This method is suitable for:

1 Preventive measures to stop contractures.

2 In serial stages to stretch a contracture.
For children, as a preventive to contracture, a preformed plastazote cylinder may be used.

Dynamic splintage on a 3-point fixation may be made. This method is used when stretch is needed (Fig. 23.6).

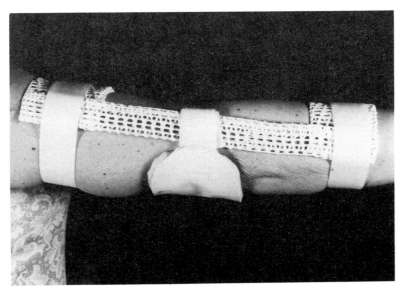

Fig. 23.6   Hexcelite elbow splint

Construction

The dynamic elbow splint is made in 5 parts (Fig. 23.7):

1 2 cuffs of Hexcelite are made to fit on the flexor aspect of the upper arm and on the forearm, in width half the circumference of the arm (A and B).
2 2 bars to join the cuffs are made from 15 cm (6 in) wide Hexcelite rolled on itself. These bars may need further reinforcing with further strips of Hexcelite or by inserting plastic-coated coat-hanger wire in the centre of the Hexcelite (C).
3 A pad made from leatherette fits over the back of the elbow joint: 1–2.5 cm (0.5–1 in) elastic straps are sewn to the pad at the sides and attached to the side bars with Velcro, fixing the Velcro to give adjustment, if necessary (D).

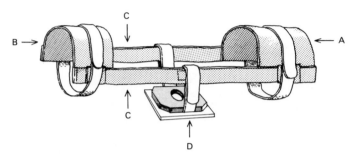

Fig. 23.7   Pattern for elbow splint

To avoid any pressure on the elbow the pad should be very well padded or made with a hole to fit over the olecranon, similar to a corn plaster.

To make the splint static rather than dynamic, non-stretch webbing straps may be substituted for the elastic.

Fastening

Crepe is bandaged over the cuffs.

Knee

Similar methods may be used on the knee.

Wrist

Splinting to maintain the wrist in a neutral position or to 30° extension is necessary for the following:
1 Burn on the volar surface of the wrist.
2 Elevation of the arm to prevent oedema may make it difficult for the unco-operative patient to extend his wrist and therefore he may develop wrist drop.
A simple wrist cock-up design is made.

Construction

A pattern is drawn and cut out from Sansplint XR or allied material (Fig. 23.8).

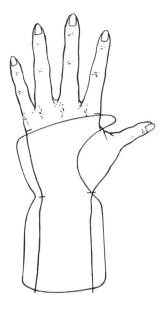

Fig. 23.8 Pattern for wrist splint

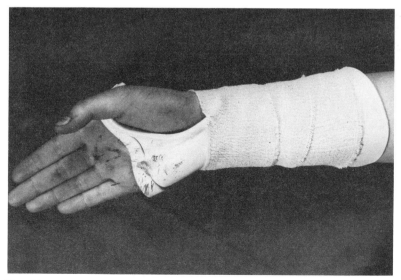

Fig. 23.9 Wrist splint

The material is cut out, heated and moulded as illustrated in Fig. 23.9. The material on the distal border and that around the thenar eminence is rolled back on itself to give increased strength and a more comfortable edge.

Care it taken that the distal border does not extend beyond the palmar crease, restricting finger movement.

Hands

Burns of the hands, particularly when full-thickness, need careful positioning to avoid deformity while healing. This necessitates splinting and is an area where particular care is taken not only in making a well-fitting splint, but also in maintaining it in the correct position.

In nearly all cases, Sansplint XR, Orthoplast or Sansplint are the preferred materials because of their exact moulding properties.

Burn Involving the Dorsum of the Hand

In these patients it is imperative to achieve the position:
1 the wrist in 20° extension
2 metacarpophalangeal joints at 70° flexion
3 interphalangeal joints in full extension (Fig. 23.10).
Without this position being maintained, the hand may heal in the claw position (metacarpophalangeal joint hyperextended and proximal interphalangeal joint flexed). It is doubly important to maintain this position if damage to the extensor apparatus has occurred, or if extensor tendons are exposed by skin loss.

The position is achieved by making a paddle splint, using the pattern shown in Fig. 23.11 and moulding to hold the joint position stated above.

If polythene bags are being used to treat these patients' hands, the splint may be made on top of the bag, but care is taken to avoid stretching the bags tightly on the hand when moulding the splint, particularly when moulding round the web space of the thumb.

If dressings are used these should be very light. Bandaging should be firm over the proximal interphalangeal joints to ensure the position is held on the splint.

Children

It is often extremely difficult to maintain a conventional paddle splint on a child and it may be necessary, if skin condition permits, to make soft leatherette slings to be positioned over the proximal interphalangeal joints and slotted through the splint as shown in

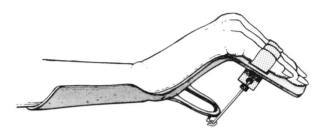

Fig. 23.10   Volar hand splint pattern

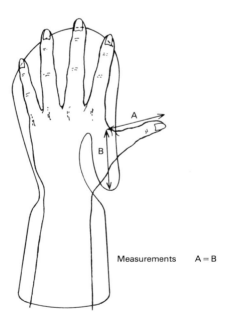

Measurements   A = B

Fig. 23.11   Volar hand splint pattern with flexor outrigger

Fig. 23.10. A small 'outrigger' may be necessary to achieve a good right-angle flexion pull. Elastic or elastic bands are used to join the slings to the splint or outrigger, using a dressmaking hook stuck to the splint with superglue.

Burns of Volar Surface

With burns involving the palm or volar surface of fingers, the aim is to maintain extension. This, initially, may be a simple static device (Fig. 23.12) with the pattern shown in Fig. 23.13, but as soon as feasible the splint should be dynamic to avoid long-term immobilization of the metacarpophalangeal joints in extension. The pattern for this is as shown in Fig. 23.14. Moulding is as shown in Fig. 23.15 and should, if stretch is to be exerted rather than just passive maintenance, be moulded close to the dorsum of the hand to the joint which is to be stretched, from which point it should be

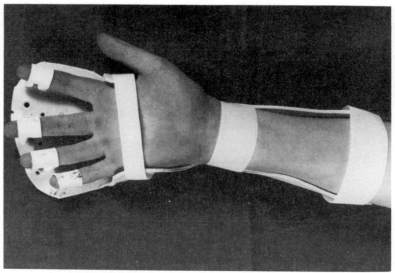

Fig. 23.12 Dorsal hand splint

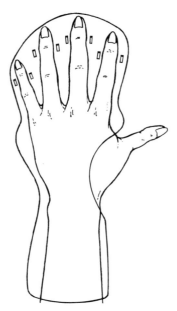

Fig. 23.13 Dorsal hand splint pattern (static)

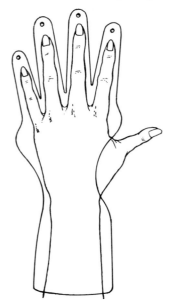

Fig. 23.14 Dorsal hand splint pattern (dynamic)

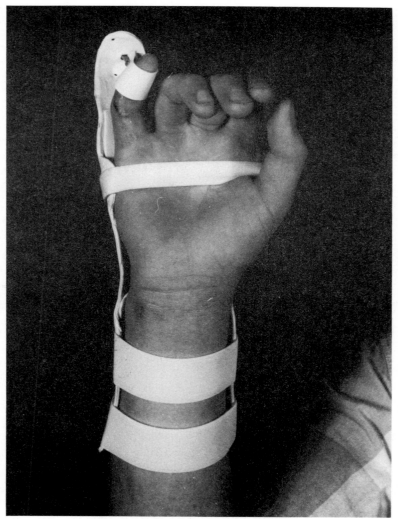

Fig. 23.15   Little finger dynamic extension splint

moulded away, as shown in Fig. 23.16. Padding is added, so that undue pressure is not exerted on the dorsum of the fingers. The slings are arranged so as to hold the fingers in extension and avoid stretching other joints unnecessarily. This splint may also be used to stretch healed but contracted skin.

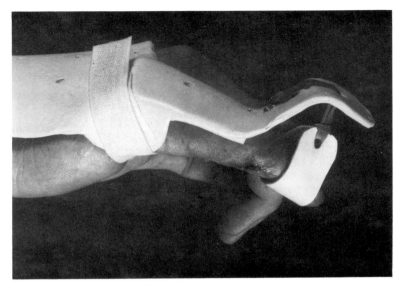

Fig. 23.16 Little finger dynamic extension splint

Children

It is often very difficult to prevent a small child from wriggling his fingers out of a dynamic extension splint. If this should be the case a static splint, as described earlier, is used or, alternatively, an *oyster splint* is made (Fig. 23.17). Hexcelite is used, as it gives better ventilation to the hand, which is completely enclosed by the splint.

Construction of an oyster splint

Two pieces of Hexcelite are cut as shown in Fig. 23.18. Measurement A is 5 cm (2 in) more than the measurement of the hand from tip of middle finger to wrist. Measurement B is the span of the hand from little finger tip to thumb tip with the fingers abducted, plus one quarter of that measurement added to each side.

To mould, the hand is placed, palm down, on a firm surface which is covered with low density 2.5 cm (1 in) foam; this in turn is covered with plastic. One piece of the Hexcelite is placed over the hand and moulding is commenced from the middle finger, working outwards to the thumb and little finger. When hard, the Hexcelite is reversed so the hand is resting in it, palm uppermost. The edges are greased to avoid adhesion with the second piece of Hexcelite which is softened and similarly moulded, this time over the palmar surface of the hand, the edges making flat contact with the edges of the first piece. To

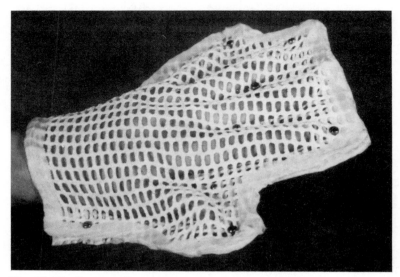

Fig. 23.17   Oyster splint

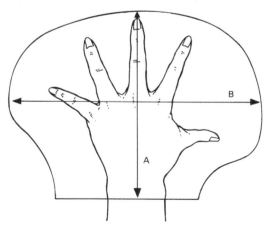

Fig. 23.18   Pattern for oyster splint

complete, stainless-steel nuts and bolts are placed at suitable positions to hold the two halves of Hexcelite together, the surplus
material is trimmed and all edges are bound with adhesive tape.

This splint needs great care in making, and in monitoring in use. It
should be removed every 2 hours to ensure no pressure areas are
being produced, sweating is not occurring within the splint, and to
exercise the fingers.

The splint is only used when other methods have proved
unsuccessful.

For burns over the whole surface of the palm and flexor aspect of the
fingers, a *'Banjo' splint* is made, as shown in Fig. 22.3 (see p.185).
The metal halo is made from 10 s w g coated mild steel, the diameter
measurements varying between 16.5 cm (6.5 in) for a small child's
hand to 24 cm (9.5 in) for an adult. The metal rings, which are spot
welded to the halo at 4 cm (1.5 in) intervals, are made from 6 mm
($\frac{5}{16}$ in) washers. The ends of the halo are attached to the patient's
wrist with plaster of Paris which extends above the elbow (the elbow
in 90° flexion). The fingers are held in extension by elastic or elastic
bands attached to the fingers by nylon sutures through the finger
nails or by sticking small pieces of leather to the nails with superglue.
These are made slightly longer than the nail, so a hole can be
punched in the leather for attachment of the elastic.

Ankle

The patient who is unable to dorsiflex his foot needs a footdrop
splint (Fig. 23.19). If the patient can actively move his ankle, he is
encouraged to do so; splinting is used when no voluntary movement
is possible, where full active dorsiflexion is not being achieved, or
when post-grafting immobilization is necessary.

The splint is made from double-thickness Hexcelite to the pattern
shown in Fig. 23.20. Measurement A = length of sole of
foot. Measurement B = angle of heel to desired length up back of
leg. Cuts are made in the material between points C and D on each
side and, while the Hexcelite is moulded to the patient's foot and leg,
points C and D are overlapped on each other and bonded to form the
heel shape.

The splint is very well padded to prevent pressure areas, particularly round the back of the heel. If required, a hole can be cut in the
Hexcelite at the back of the heel.

Allowance is made for the padding when measuring and moulding
to the patient's leg.

An anti-roll bar may be fitted to the back of the ankle portion of
the splint to prevent external rotation of the leg.

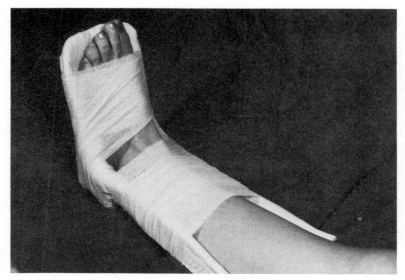

Fig. 23.19   Ankle splint

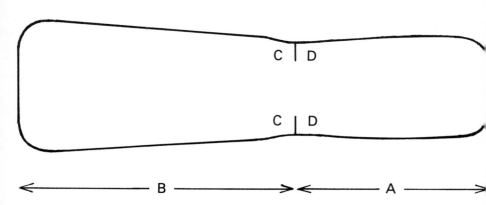

Fig. 23.20   Ankle splint pattern

Suppliers

San Splint XR	Smith and Nephew Ltd PO Box 81, Hessle Road Hull HU3 2BN Tel: 0482-25181
Orthoplast	Johnson & Johnson Brunel Way, Slough SL1 4XR Tel: 0753-32134
Hexcelite	Orthopaedic Systems Unit G22 Oldgate St Michaels Industrial Estate Widnes, Cheshire WA8 8TL Tel: 051-420 3250/6409
Aquaplast	Camp Therapy Northgate House Staple Gardens Winchester, Hampshire Tel: 0962-55248
Orfit	Seton Orthopaedics Tubiton House Medlock Street Oldham, Lancashire OL1 3HS Tel: 061-652 2222
Leatherette	DIY shops, upholstery shops
Pneumatic collars	Surgical Fitters, Gilbert & Mellish 499/504 Bristol Road Birmingham B29 6AU Tel: 021-471 3055
Suspan heating pan	Hinders Leslies Ltd Green Pond Road, London E17 6EN Tel: 01-531 4100
Adhesive foams	Seton Orthopaedics Tubiton House, Medlock Street, Oldham, Lancashire OL1 3HS Tel: 061-652 2222 and Hinders Leslies Ltd Green Pond Road, London E17 6EN Tel: 01-531 4100

References

BARR, R.N.(1975) *The Hand: Principles and Techniques of Splint Making.* Butterworths, London.

EVANS, E.B., LARSON, D.L. & YATES, S. (1968) Preservation and Restoration of Joint Function in Patients with Severe Burns. *J. Am. Med. Assoc.*, **204**, 91.

FESS, E., GETTLE, K. STRICKLAND, (1981) *Hand Splinting, Principles and Methods.* C.V. Mosby, St. Louis.

FISHER, S. & HELM, P. (1984) *Comprehensive Rehabilitation of Burns.* Williams and Wilkins, Baltimore.

FOWLER, D. & PEGG, S.P.(1983) Evaluation of Aquaplast Splinting in a Burns Unit. *Burns, 9*, 284.

MALICK, M.H. (1975) Management of the Severely Burned Patient. *Br. J. Occup. Ther.*, **38**, 76.

MALICK, M.H. (1976) *Manual on Static Hand Splinting.* Harmaville Rehabilitation Center, Pittsburg, Pa, 15238.

MALICK, M.H. (1978) *Manual of Dynamic Hand Splinting with Thermoplastic materials.* Harmaville Rehabilitation Centre, Pittsburg, Pa, 15238.

MALICK, M.H. & CARR, J.A.(1982) *Manual on Management of the Burn Patient.* Harmaville Rehabilitation Center, Pittsburg, Pa, 15238.

(The above three manuals are available from Camp Ltd., Northgate House, Staple Gardens, Winchester SO23 8ST. UK)

MOBERG, E. (1984) *Splinting in Hand Therapy.* G. Thieme, Stuttgart.

VAN-STRATEN, O. & MAHLER, D.(1981) Hexcelite Splints for Burned and Traumatised Hand. *Burns, 8*, 188.

24

The Burns Team and Unit

The Multidisciplinary Team

Expert care of a patient with major burn injury requires many specialized skills from a large multidisciplinary team, which includes:

1 Plastic surgeons, physicians, paediatricians, psychiatrists and psychologists.
2 Nurses, physiotherapsts and occupational therapists experienced in intensive care work, plastic surgical techniques, paediatric, geriatric and psychiatric care, and operating theatre skills.
3 Dietician, social worker, secretaries, domestics, porters and hospital chaplains who all require knowledge of the special needs of burn injured patients.
4 Personnel working in the support services such as biochemistry, microbiology, central sterile supplies, laundry and pharmacy, also need to be aware of the special requirements in provision of critical burn care.

The dramatic effect of severe burn injury on the human body, both physical and psychological, and the close team work involved in critical care, create a very stressful working environment. Therefore the selection of staff includes assessment of ability to:

1 cope with personal stress,
2 work compatibly with other members of the team,
3 provide emotional support for colleagues as well as patients.

Some of the advantages of treating burn injured patients in a burn centre are that:

1 Staff acquire expertise in this very specialized field by continuous experience.
2 The team is large enough to provide group support.

The work in the burns unit involves expertise from many specialities which include:

1 Accident and emergency care: because the patient's condition frequently deteriorates after the first few hours post-injury,

211

resuscitation may be intense and prolonged. Therefore on admission to the burns unit the patient requires continuation of the emergency resuscitation and treatment commenced in the accident and emergency department. Emergency surgery such as escharotomy may also be required (see page 36).

2 Critical care: Even after initial improvement has been sustained for many days relapses are common, especially following essential surgery to regain skin cover. Many operations may be required before skin closure is complete; therefore recurrent crises are a predominant feature of major burn illness.

3 Plastic surgery: The techniques required for closure of extensive skin defects and subsequent reconstruction of burn damaged tissues involve the extensive use of grafts and flaps.

4 Paediatric care: approximately 50% of all major burn injuries occur in children. A severely burnt child is likely to remain a patient of the plastic surgery and burn centre until he is adult, requiring many reconstructive operations during his growth and development. Therefore the importance of gaining the child's confidence and co-operation from the first admission cannot be overstressed.

5 Care of the elderly: Even quite small percentage burns result in critical illness in the elderly, who on recovery from the acute phase require intensive and prolonged rehabilitation to regain function and self confidence. A clear understanding of the specific problems and needs of the elderly is essential for successful rehabilitation.

6 Terminal care: Some victims of major burn have no hope of survival, but may survive the initial injury and live for a few days. Once a patient has been expertly assessed and found to be terminally ill all further resuscitation measures will merely prolong the terminal illness by a few more days. Therefore treatment is aimed at the relief of pain, general comfort of the patient, and the provision of counselling and emotional support for his relatives and friends.

7 Control of infection: infection is the major cause of mortality and morbidity in burn-injured patients. A thorough knowledge of microbiology and the clinical manifestations of various infections is essential for early detection and treatment of the infected burn victim, and for the prevention of cross infection.

The Nursing Team in the Burns Unit

As the largest single work force and the personnel who provide continuous 24 hour care for the critically injured patient, a highly skilled and well co-ordinated nursing team is paramount.

The mixture of male/female, age group and experience all need to be taken into account in selection of staff.

Because burn care frequently requires a long stay in an enclosed unit the team require expertise in multiple aspects of nursing in order to provide appropriate care to all patients throughout their admission. For example:

1 A large minority of critical burn injuries occur in children.

2 Because of their reduced mobility, disabled and elderly people are prone to severe burn injuries, most commonly scalding accidents. The older the patient the more critical his burn illness (see page 5) and more prolonged his rehabilitation.

3 In recent years suicide by self-inflicted burns has become more prevalent.

4 Assault by burning has increased.

5 There has been an increase in the number of burn injuries as a result of intoxication with alcohol or drugs.

6 The number of domestic and industrial accidents resulting in burn injuries has decreased.

As a result of these changes in the type of burn victim requiring care, the burns unit tends to have patients who are mostly very young or elderly. Of the young adult and middle-aged patients many suffer from mental illness, alcoholism or drug addiction.

The varied experience of the nursing team should reflect a balance between the various special skills likely to be required.

Many nurses on first caring for a victim of major burn injury find they are faced with unprecedented emotional stress. For example:

1 It is a common phenomenon in major burn injuries that the patient's condition steadily deteriorates over the first week following injury. Despite the most intensive and skilled treatment the patient who is conscious, well orientated and well motivated on admission, after a few days may be unconscious, unresponsive and requiring artificial ventilation.

2 The difficulties in counselling and offering emotional support to the patient, his relatives and friends in such circumstances are obvious.

3 The burn wounds may look relatively innocuous on admission but over the next few days become horrific in appearance and smell foul.

4 Compared to other types of wound care, redressing major burn wounds is a marathon. The nurse may find it difficult to imagine the enormity of the task until she assists with the dressing procedure. Many nurses admit to a feeling of panic on first seeing the extent of the wound and the amount of dressing material requiring application before the patient is comfortable again. If the patient is conscious the nurse's stress is heightened by the patient's distress at the sight and smell of his wounds. If the patient is also

critically ill there is additional anxiety about how the patient's emotional stress is affecting his physically precarious condition.

5 Nurses frequently complain that even after leaving the burns unit, taking a shower and washing their hair, they can still smell the burn victim's wounds for hours.

Caring for critically ill patients requires intense concentration. Add to this the counselling of very distressed relatives, the sight and smell of burn wounds and working in an uncomfortably warm and humid environment one can readily understand why nurses find this type of work extremely tiring both physically and mentally. It is not unusual for nurses to show early signs of stress by recurrent nightmares, often related to fire.

The Burns Unit

The ideal burns unit is purpose built to allow complete control over the physical environment.

Heating

Since body temperature control can be a major problem for the burn-injured patient, it is necessary to change rapidly the temperature of the environment for individual patients between a range of 20°–27°C. (68°–80°F). Humidity remains between 30 and 60% RH depending on room temperature.

Control of Infection

Infection in burns is a major cause of mortality; therefore all critically burnt patients require isolation in a single room which is fully equipped for reverse barrier nursing and barrier nursing.

Positive pressure ventilation in patient's rooms may assist in preventing infection being carried into the room in reverse barrier nursing, but increases the risk of spreading infection when barrier nursing is required. Therefore the ideal situation would allow positive pressure ventilation when required to be converted into normal or negative pressure ventilation where infection is established. In practice the engineering to achieve this is so complex and expensive that a compromise is inevitable.

Air conditioning throughout a burns unit should be designed to ensure an air flow pattern from the 'sterile' areas, such as theatre, treatment and patient rooms, to 'less sterile' areas, such as sluice, annexes and corridors.

Terminal filters are required to filter out dust particles which may carry bacteria.

Space

The theatre, treatment room and patient rooms must be large enough to allow many staff access to the patient at one time, and permit the use of a lot of equipment, e.g. electronic monitoring machines, drip regulators, ventilators, and haemodialysis equipment.

Staff require easy access to a drink dispensing machine when working in very high room temperatures, and a comfortable rest room which is private from the clinical environment.

Interior Design

The interior design of the burns unit should take into account the following:

1 *Decor*
   (a) Considerable stresses are placed on patients and staff in a burns unit; therefore the decor should be peaceful.
   (b) Burn injured patients tend to feel persistently cold, therefore soft warm colours are preferred.
2 *Light*
   (a) Essential observations of the patient include colour of the normal and injured skin. Room lighting should not distort natural skin tones.
   (b) Some dressing procedures are very delicate and require 'theatre standard' lighting.
   (c) Patients with burns to and around the eyes are more comfortable in soft lighting.
3 *Communications*
   (a) A good visual and verbal communication system is essential both during the critical illness and when the patient is being 'weaned off specialling'.
   (b) Constant surveillance of the patient may be essential for many weeks and can be greatly assisted by closed circuit television.
   (c) For the patient who is in a single room and trying to re-establish his identity the need for an excellent verbal communication system with those caring for him and with the 'outside world' cannot be over-emphasized. An internal communication system and British Telecom telephone link should be available and usable by patients who cannot use their hands.

The Burns Theatre

In surgical terms all burns must be considered infected. Therefore a theatre designated solely for the treatment of burns is highly desirable.

Because of the critical condition of many burnt patients undergoing surgery the theatre is best sited within or adjacent to the burns unit.

Sufficient space is required to permit three or four surgeons and their assistants access to the patient and allow room for a large volume of equipment. For the critically ill patient speed in completion of extensive surgery may be life saving, hence the practice of using up to four surgeons at one time. Time wasted in waiting for access to the patient may hazard the patient's chance of survival.

Large amounts of equipment must be readily available and well maintained. Storage space should take account of the unusually large quantity of dressings and fluids required for a single patient.

Location of the Burns Unit

Care of the burn injured patient is an extension of the plastic surgery speciality, and it is beneficial for both patients and staff if the burns unit is sited in close proximity to a plastic surgery centre.

Burns units tend to suffer great fluctuations in work load and therefore are assisted in excessively busy times by the availability of extra personnel from a plastic surgery centre, who have the basic skills required to assist adequately the burns unit team.

After intensive and often lengthy treatment in the enclosed atmosphere of the burns unit, the patient who is extensively burnt may benefit from transfer to a plastic surgery ward during the convalescent phase of his illness.

Following initial recovery from critical illness the burnt patient and his family may have to come to terms with the fact that he is disfigured and will need repeated admission to the plastic surgery centre for reconstructive surgery over many months or years before his recovery is complete. Even after extensive reconstructive surgery the patient with severe burn scars may be left with permanent disfigurement. The opportunity in the plastic surgery centre to meet others who suffer similar disfigurement, and who have had surgery to improve the function of their limbs and their appearance, assists the patient who is still shocked and depressed by his new appearance.

Staff working in the plastic surgery specialty are experienced in caring for disfigured people and use the opportunities available to continue the work of the burn care team in counselling the patient and his family. They encourage ex-burn patients to assist the newly disfigured in re-establishing his identity and coming to terms with his new body image.

Good communication between the burn unit staff and plastic surgery centre staff is essential in maintaining continuity of care. During the critical stage of his illness the burn-injured patient becomes dependent on the burns unit team. Therefore the close proximity of the burns unit and plastic surgery centre enable those staff whom the patient has come to rely upon to visit him and help him gain confidence in the new team continuing his care.

Good liaison also ensures that all staff are familiar with the rapid developments currently occurring in all aspects of the treatment and aftercare of the victims of major burn injury.

References

LAING, J.E. (1966) Design of a New Burns Unit. In *Research in Burns*, ed. Wallace and Wilkinson. Churchill Livingstone, Edinburgh.

LOWBURY, E.J.L. (1954) Air Conditioning for Filtered Air for Dressing Burns. *Lancet*, **i**, 292.

LOWBURY, E.J.L. (1975) Recent Studies in the Control of Burn Infections. *Burns*, **2**, 26.

MCGREGOR, J.C., SUTHERLAND, A.B. *et al.* (1981) Are Expensive and Elaborate Burns Units always Necessary? *Burns*, **7**, 166.

TAIT, B.M. & RUSSELL, J. (1970) Aspects of Nursing in a Burns Unit. *3rd Int. Congr. Research in Burns, Abstracts*, Prague p.255.

WILKINS, T.J. & CAMPBELL, J.L. (1981) Psychosocial Concerns in a Paediatric Burn Unit. *Burns*, **7**, 208.

WORMOLD, P.J. (1970) Effect of a Changed Environment on Bacteria Colonisation Rates in a Burns Unit. *J. Hygiene (Camb.)*, **68**, 633.

25

Psychiatric Aspects of Burn Injury

It is important for burn surgeons to have some understanding of the psychological problems of the burned. Patients are quick to pick up this empathy and it is likely to be a help in their recovery. The will to survive depends on many things and a patient's awareness that his problems are understood in more than a technical sense is of considerable help.

Burned patients are not a random sample of population; burned children may come from disorganized homes with parents who have personal or psychiatric difficulties. In adults a larger population than expected have pre-existing mental illness such as depression, schizophrenia, drug dependence, alcoholism or dementia.

The stress of thermal injury may induce acute psychological reactions which produce management problems and complicate recovery.

In spite of success in the first weeks of treatment in the supportive but unreal world of the burns unit, the patient has to face not only the continuing problems of his personal health but often major life problems such as the loss of loved ones or colleagues in a fire, loss of home, inability to work, personal deformity or financial loss. It is not surprising therefore, that amongst severely burned patients a considerable proportion when followed up at one year had experienced moderate to severe psychiatric sequelae.

Burns often have medico-legal implications; serious questions of public policy, institutional management, criminal injury, negligence and personal injustice may arise. The case notes may well be subject to scrutiny by opposing interests at court. The doctor has a public duty to contribute towards social justice. Clearly written case notes which give some idea of the psychological state and degree of suffering at the time will be of help to the surgeon when compiling the legal reports that will be requested to aid the courts in securing a just settlement.

The surgeon remains the lynchpin of care but faces a psychologically delicate task remaining sensitive to the morale and efficiency of staff, alert to the patient's changing needs and those of the busy professionals who assist from time to time.

Obtaining Psychiatric and Psychological Advice

Burns and plastic surgery share with the mental health specialties a team approach, and a surgeon's skill in involving and sustaining the interest of other professionals is likely to be a useful asset. The newly arrived surgeon should find out the local referral process and with support from colleagues in the team attempt to improve or consolidate the liaison service.

Mental illness or mental health has an almost infinite extent in terms of the demand that the population can make. In most medical services, psychiatry is a shortage specialty and therefore, most professionals in it have plenty to occupy their time. A large burns unit could absorb the services of a considerable part of each week of a social worker, clinical psychologist and psychiatrist but few will have such resources available.

In the United Kingdom the realities of the financial implications of health care have recently become more apparent to doctors. In any system the long-term care of the chronically mentally ill impose enormous costs and it is for this reason that psychiatrists often work strictly in 'catchment' areas. This has the advantage of clearly defining the medical and financial responsibility for the provision of continuing care. One disadvantage is that, where burns units function on a regional health authority basis, the advising psychiatrist is unlikely to be able to undertake the continuing care of many of the burned, but at least he will know the appropriate psychiatric colleague for further referral.

Currently both psychiatry and clinical psychology remain growth areas compared with medicine and surgery and there is an increasing interest in the contribution that these services can make. Fashionably called Liaison Psychiatry it is essentially nothing new but, thus highlighted, it commands attention, more systematic study and hopefully will lead to improvement in service and training. Liaisons which are intimate relations and connections require an input from both sides to be successful.

Available Members of the Mental Health Team

At the risk of stating the obvious it might be helpful for some to delineate the functions of some members of the mental health team.

Psychiatrists

These are medical graduates who specialize in the treatment of mental illness. Like all medical graduates but unlike psychologists and social workers they can prescribe drugs. There are three main specialties: adult mental illness, child psychiatry and mental handicap.

Clinical psychologists

These are graduates in psychology (the study of normal behaviour). In addition they have spent a further three years studying aspects of mental illness to qualify in clinical psychology. Like medical graduates their skills and interests vary considerably. In general they are familiar with most forms of mental illness but are particularly skilled in the psychological management of anxiety, phobias and minor nervous reactions; they have some knowledge of behavioural and group methods of treatment and may be knowledgable on the practice and pitfalls of the measurement of human behaviour.

Mental health officers

Mental health officers are qualified social workers who have taken an approved course of study in mental illness and the law. They are concerned with the formal detention of psychiatric patients in hospital under the Mental Health Act in order that they might receive appropriate treatment. They have a duty to protect the rights of the mentally ill individual and society at large. Usually there is a 24 hours nationwide service and the local psychiatric service will know how to obtain the name and telephone number of the relevant person.

How to obtain advice

In a planned service ideally the liaison psychiatrist will visit the unit on a regular basis at a predictable time and will deal with routine and follow-up matters.

There are also likely to be less regular urgent consultations whenever time can be found. If a consultation is really urgent insist on personal communication with the psychiatrist to stress the nature and urgency of the problem. Distillation of contact through one or two secretaries may have unfortunate results. Although for routine referrals personal contact is desirable, where it is possible a written referral slip according to local practice may still be useful for the psychiatrist's own records.

In the absence of the planned service, the local psychiatric hospital is likely to have a 24 hour duty psychiatrist with consultant support. The local senior psychiatric nursing officer may be able to advise concerning difficult nursing problems. Many services have community psychiatric nurses often of charge nurse, or sister grade on 24 hour call and they may be available to visit in an emergency.

Detention under the Mental Health Act

These laws are designed to protect the mentally ill individual, and society from the mentally ill. The technicalities need not concern the trainee burn surgeon. It will suffice to say that under common law in an emergency the doctor is required to act in the patient's best interest and common sense is the best guide. The presence of certification under the Mental Health Act is no barrier to treatment in a burns unit. The absence of certification in a mentally deranged unco-operative patient in a less urgent setting may be more of a problem and the psychiatric service of the referring agency should be able to advise. Your local psychiatrist and mental health officer will be familiar with the sections of the Mental Health Act in common usage and have access to information on the rarer ones in use.

Problems of Consent to Treatment in the Mentally Ill

For the transiently confused or the chronically demented, the surgeon should try to convey the essence of the proposed treatment at an appropriate time and secure the consent of a relative when practical. On rare occasions there are some mentally ill patients with a degree of insight who refuse to co-operate with treatment and local expert psychiatric advice on how to proceed should be obtained. The patient confronted with a united front from surgical, psychiatric and nursing staff usually complies. However, on some occasions formal certification is appropriate and this is of considerable help to the nursing staff who may have to administer the unwanted treatment.

Psychiatric Aspects of the Patient which Contribute to the Burn Injury

The psychiatrically disturbed are at relatively high risk for thermal injury for reasons which are largely self evident.

Almost the entire range of major psychiatric diagnoses may be encountered at some time in a burns unit. Both extremes of age are well represented. Babies and children will be discussed in a later section; the elderly with a multiplicity of psychological, physical and sometimes psychiatric handicaps are well represented.

Psychological and Psychiatric Aspects during Hospital Stay

The commonest alerting feature is the nature of the action leading to the burn injury. There have been various studies analysing the presence and attempting to predict the likelihood of psychiatric complications whilst in hospital and after discharge. The patient groups are heterogeneous but three important factors emerge as predictors.

1 A history of existing or past psychiatric illness.
2 The age of the patient, delirious states being commoner with increasing age, and
3 More controversially, the severity of the burn injury.

Management of Existing Psychiatric Disorders

On admission to the unit the immediate burns management takes priority. Apart from the very rare occasions when there is an obvious psychiatric emergency as well, there is usually time to obtain information about the present and past psychiatric history. Many chronically psychotic patients when suffering from a serious acute physical ailment show a surprising improvement in their level of awareness even if it is transient. Likewise the chronically anxious, nervous and obsessional usually cope well for a while.

Should psychotropic drugs be continued?

If the burn is mild and little anaesthesia or active surgical treatment is required, then probably the psychotropic drugs should continue. If the burn is not in this category and there is a likelihood of anaesthesia and surgical procedures being required for the burn, then it is probably safer to withhold antidepressant and major tranquillizers until psychiatric advice can be obtained. Very few patients will relapse into profound psychotic states if drugs are discontinued for a few days.

Problems of drug dependence

Exceptions to the above advice include benzodiazepines, drugs used in narcotic addiction, anticonvulsants, lithium and the commonly self-prescribed drug alcohol. Withdrawal symptoms from the cessation of minor tranquillizers are not uncommon and could add to the patient's distress and discomfort; occasionally reactions are severe. The better recognized symptoms and signs associated with narcotic drug dependence are often not as severe as expected and are amenable to control with minor or major tranquillizers in reducing dosage over several days.

Lithium salts

These are used as a prophylactic drug in the management of manic depressive psychosis. Sudden withdrawal has been associated with lapse into hypomania or depression. In established cases under treatment, regular blood tests are used to monitor a therapeutic level. Too low a level is ineffective and too high dangerous. If renal function is impaired then the drug can only be used with extreme caution. Thus a patient on lithium requires urgent expert psychiatric advice on the balance of risk of continuance versus withdrawal of the drug.

Alcohol

Alcoholism is still commonly missed. Few patients volunteer their dependence and relatives are sometimes reluctant to add to the potential problems faced by the burns team. There may be clues in the circumstances of the burn, occupation, appearance and clinical signs. A probing and detailed history from a relative or close friend is probably the best guide. The sudden withdrawal of alcohol may produce epileptic fits, severe shakiness and restlessness merging into delirium tremens.

Psychological and Psychiatric Problems Developing in Burns Care

Organic psychoses are not uncommon especially delirium from a variety of causes and particularly alcoholic delirium tremens which merits special description. A variety of depressive disorders may present and also drug-withdrawal states. Psychologically there are the problems of coping with physical handicap, deformity and disfigurement, approaching death and fear of it and, for some, bereavement, loss of home and employment.

Delirium

This is characterized by the recent onset of clouding of consciousness, disorientation, impaired attention and memory, agitation, motor restlessness and sometimes hallucinations and transient delusions. In burns units such states usually occur within the first month. There are a multiplicity of possible organic causes and attempts should be made to treat the cause where possible, e.g. infection, anoxia, sleep deprivation and cardiac failure. The elderly are more prone to delirium. If necessary tranquillizing drugs such as haloperidol and chlorpromazine may be given. The regular encouragement and recognition of patients by nursing staff, daily identification of reality and conversation in more rational moments are helpful. Explanation and support for and by relatives is a useful adjunct.

Alcoholic delirium

Alcoholic delirium is discussed separately as it is not uncommon, is particularly dangerous and, in view of possible alcohol-withdrawal epileptic fits, it is treated slightly differently. Typically it comes on three to four days after withdrawal with a range of one to ten days. Patients are extremely frightened, intermittently confused and disorientated and often visually hallucinated seeing small unpleasant animals and objects. In this irrational state they are likely to be uncooperative and potentially violent. Even without burns it has a generally quoted mortality of around 15%. The requirements are to predict whether this state might occur and to prescribe prophylactic sedative drugs; if it has occurred to act swiftly and effectively. Experts vary on specific drug treatment but there is general agreement that chlordiazepoxide, diazepam, chlormethiazole and haloperidol are all effective given in moderately large doses decreasing over several days. (See *Treatment of Violent Patients* p.230.) Fluid replacement, B vitamins and special nursing measures are important. The other widespread pathological effects of alcohol on the body and mind should be remembered and appropriately treated.

Drug withdrawal states

These have been described above. Hidden barbiturate dependence is now less common but withdrawal fits can occur.

Depression during burns recovery

Many authors comment that depression occurs frequently. The term can be loosely used and can cover admission to periods of sombre reflection, months of mild loss of drive and enthusiasm, bouts of emotionally charged anguish through to prolonged stuporosed, retarded psychotic states. Remember that some individuals conceal their emotional feelings and others display them relatively easily. Paradoxically, as burns care becomes more sophisticated, some successful survivors will have far greater psychological as well as physical handicaps to face.

Thus depression lasting a few days may commonly be seen within the unit. It is to be expected, should be recognized and when appropriate discussed. Drug treatment is unnecessary and undesirable. More serious depression affecting ability to eat and sleep and the will to recover will need more detailed assessment. Individuals may have much guilt about their predicament and perhaps others involved in the precipitating incident. It may be necessary to suggest to the more reticent that they feel low or down enabling them to start to discuss their feelings. In such cases do not be frightened to ask about their feelings about the future and suicide. There is no need to fear that the doctor is implanting such ideas within the patient and many are very relieved to be able to discuss them. If these enquiries are positive then ask about whether any plans or methods have been conceived. If as is likely further psychiatric advice is to be obtained explain your referral to the patient. In these cases there is no need to start immediatly on antidepressant drugs; wait until a fuller assessment has been made.

During outpatient follow up, if moderate or serious depression is manifest, it will probably be better to alert the psychiatric service near to where the patient is living as treatment may take months and one is more likely to achieve a continuity of care in this setting.

Coping with physical handicap deformity and disfigurement

Depending upon the site and extent of the injury and the individual's constitution and maturity, there is likely to be a range of emotional reactions including anger, frustration and despair. Patients will need explanation about the short-term effects of burns and inflammatory swelling. To the newly arrived patient facial oedema and eyelid swelling may seem more important than a full-thickness burn to a limb. Beauty of appearance though more highly prized in women than in men is of psychological importance to both and the disfigurement caused by facial burns is often a severe, profound and long-lasting handicap. Psychologically the face has a significance far beyond its proportionate surface area. Traditionally society expects a stoical attitude to affliction and such an attitude is convenient to the surgical and nursing staff sparing them to a degree from the suffering of others. On the other hand there is some evidence that psychological intervention by discussion and explanation of the difficulties leads to better adaptation.

Non-survivable burns and approaching death

Though doctors are usually dispassionate and professional about the statistical chances of death, generally our handling of the psychological needs of those about to die are poorly developed. Imbus and Zawacki faced the problem squarely and point out that there is a considerable difference between saying a case is hopeless and that survival is unprecedented. In, say, a 90% major burn, the survivor may only have a few hours of clarity of thought left and in that precious time they discussed the outlook dispassionately with their

patients. Some opted for 'ordinary care' rather than 'a full therapeutic regime'. Whenever there was doubt the latter course was
adopted.

It is important for the patient, loved ones and relatives to be able to
say goodby albeit often by indirect reference. There should be room
for relatives to express their grief. Such grief should be actively
recognized by surgeons and staff. If all possible has been done and
dignity preserved relatives can then take comfort as they see the staff
continue with their care for others.

Psychological Support in Hospital and after Discharge

This is a problem in all health services as there is conflict between
patient demand, the clinical need and the resources available. The
best that can be advocated is for the surgeon to draw up a series of
strategic guidelines.

1 Assess the clinical need for support.
2 Consider and acknowledge, shape and where necessary encourage
  the present support within the burns team.
3 Look around the unit and the follow-up arrangements to see,
  including oneself, who might be available to help in a constructive
  manner and decide roughly how long it should be sustained.
4 Identify those areas where highly skilled professional help is
  essential and secure it (surgical, psychiatric, physiotherapeutic
  etc.).
5 Be aware of the emotional support (or lack of it) from other
  patients.
6 Consider introduction to various self help groups.
7 Write your plan clearly in a typed script perhaps in the summary
  or a letter to the general practitioner so that it is clear to others as
  well as yourself.
8 Expect to modify the plans as problems emerge or subside. Make
  time to listen to the patient's real life difficulties.

If resources are stretched and scarce in the affluent western world
spare a thought for the bulk of the world population. Throughout
history most patients have a remarkable tolerance for lack of
resources but not for cursory dismissal. Self help groups as well as
being therapeutic can become politically helpful in allocating more
resources to the problems of the burned.

According to case notes, reassurance is a commodity liberally
dispensed but sometimes it is merely a cover for hurried doctors
with deaf ears and in this setting it is little help to either. Patients are

reassured if they feel that the doctors and staff have a comprehensive understanding of their difficulties and are knowledgeable within their own speciality. Whilst not wishing to understate the horrific and vast problems that some individuals have to overcome it is surprising how often apparently overwhelming problems do sort themselves out over time. Support and encouragement need to be given in the interim.

Where patient dissatisfaction appears inappropriate to the level of disability, discussion with a close relative or a conversation with the patient's general practitioner (if he is known to him) may be quite revealing. Occasionally psychiatric consultation may be helpful. However, some patients feel threatened by such a suggestion believing that insanity or dishonesty is imputed and when they present to the psychiatrist with a firm face of normality and reasonableness it can be difficult to penetrate the facade. It is therefore, necessary to try and explain beforehand the links between physical morbidity, emotion and psychological function.

Psychiatric Aspects of the Family of Burned Patients

The most important variable is the age of the patient. Thus the family problems faced in infancy, childhood and adolescence are all very different concerning development, maturation, schooling and work training. In adult life the focus shifts to parenthood, financial solvency, social consequences of increasing infirmity and senility and coping with the concomitant increasing personality and intellectual rigidity. Certain general factors can be dealt with.

Anxiety about the Immediate Outcome

It is easy for busy professionals to forget that the average person has only the remotest idea about the course and outcome of burns care. Families stressed by the burn incident, perhaps involved in it or partly to blame may have difficulty in grasping the significance of the advice given. Information that the mind does not want to hear is sometimes totally repressed or the intellectual message though encoded fails to penetrate to emotional significance. Thus there is sometimes a need to repeat the information at spaced intervals to enable families to grasp the realistic situation. How this is done will vary from unit to unit but frequent visiting and contact with the burns team members is likely to be the usual method. For certain cases more specific and individual plans may need to be made. Fears about the deformity at present and in the future and the ability of relatives to handle it are common.

Guilt

Guilt is common. Much of it may be entirely understandable, perhaps a mother not supervising her child, an unfaithful spouse precipitating a suicide attempt, a daughter not supervising her demented mother. Commonly though the guilt is less easily apportioned.

Some guilt is grossly disporportionate and if persistent then further investigation into the circumstances and the psychopathology of the individual will be warranted.

Projection of anger and guilt

Sometimes these emotions instead of being resolved internally are pushed outwards towards the medical and other staff. It is fairly easy to find faults in any complex system of care and whereas lack of resources may be defensible, unsatisfactory staff attitudes are not. There are times when recognition of this projective mechanism may be useful. On the other hand being aware of our imperfections it should not be freely invoked. Although professionally even-handed and egalitarian in our care, there may be some families and relatives that will require extra consideration and it is well worth giving time and thought at an early stage rather than being involved months later in hours of painstaking investigation of notes, individuals and fading memories with a sometimes fruitless outcome to all concerned.

Active involvement of the family

As much burn care is protracted, active involvement of the family can be very useful from an early stage. At first details of the history, background and personality may be obtained. Support and encouragement is given by the family by visiting and perhaps extending their involvement to others less fortunate. They may also be valuable in active reinforcement of rehabilitative aims.

Psychiatric and Psychological Aspects for Nursing and Paramedical Staff

Psychiatric Illness in the Patient

As for surgical staff, this presents another complicating variable in the patient's management. Staff may have little or no experience in the management of the mentally ill, staff anxiety levels may be raised, there may be fears of uncertainty, violence, how to cope with non-compliance and irrationality and difficulty in establishing rapport. The devolvement of psychiatric experience to all nurses in training lessens this problem and some burns units make a point of having some senior staff with psychiatric qualifications. Psychiatric referral may be helpful particularly in potentially explosive situations as the problems can be assessed well before difficulties arise.

Stress among staff

Most staff enjoy the excitement, responsibility and team work of surgical and burns treatment. Exceptionally a few will find it particularly stressful and good management will identify this and take appropriate action. The adage 'one man's meat is another man's poison' receives some experimental support in the study of the personalities of trained nurses choosing to work in intensive care. Some people thrive in what to others appear anxiety-provoking conditions. Students and trainees have less option but may be relieved by limit of time. If there are problems of high sickness rates, low morale and individual breakdown then a closer look at the unit organization and that individual's personal circumstances will be more fruitful than blaming the nature of the work.

Joint discussion

Many burns teams have formalized rounds and meetings to discuss patient care, long-term outcome and death and it is important that the disciplines contributing in this process have a chance to participate actively. Where burns are treated on a surgical ward as an occasional procedure it is important for the surgeon to set up such a forum for discussion and not only at the bedside.

Management of the Violent Burned Patient

A violent patient is not only a danger to himself but to the welfare of other patients and staff. Violence produces high anxiety levels in staff unaccustomed to dealing with it; decision making, judgement and concentration may be impaired; prompt management is required.

Ideally, potential violence should be predicted and prevented. A detailed history from relatives and observers can highlight potential problem areas.

Where possible talk, patience, understanding and skilled nursing care may settle the patient.

At other times a combination of physical restraint and medication may be required depending on the clinical condition of the burned patient and the aetiology of the violence. Again ideally one should know the nature of the condition causing the violence prior to any drug treatment or at least have a good indication of the cause.

Once calmness has been restored there should be a careful review of the patient's condition to ensure that the aetiology is understood and is correct and predictions made as to the likelihood of further violence and plans for its control. Seek specialist advice and help when necessary.

Occasionally there is continuing violence or difficult behaviour. Most organic delirious states are of relatively short duration but a few chronically mentally ill patients can present continuing nursing difficulties even in the most skilled hands. Such individuals are likely to be known to their psychiatric service and it may be useful to explore with them what help they can offer with both advice and detachment of nursing personnel. Alternatively if they are remote from the surgical unit, the local psychiatric service or temporary psychiatric nursing support may be of value.

Likely Causes of Violence in the Burns Unit

1 Organic delirium, the features of which have been described above of which alcoholic delirium is a special sub-category. Other causes may include septicaemia, anoxia, metabolic and drug withdrawal states (pp.222–224).
2 Functional psychoses, usually with a pre-existing history of schizophrenia or occasionally the manic phase of a manic depressive psychosis.
3 Occasional personality disorders reacting to stress.

Drug Treatment

The general principles of drug administration must be upheld concerning dose compared with body weight, extremes of age, other conditions and treatments. Where there is thought to be a risk of withdrawal epileptic fits, chlormethiazole or chlordiazepoxide (both of which have anticonvulsant properties) are to be preferred.

Chlormethiazole is commonly administered by capsule 0.2 g, or syrup 0.25 g in 5 ml. Depending on the condition two to four capsules can be given immediately and repeated within a few hours. An intravenous preparation given over the course of ten minutes is available but this is sometimes impractical in the circumstances.

Chlordiazepoxide can be given orally and intramuscularly 25–100 mg and repeated two to four hourly up to a maximum of 400 mg per day.

Of the major tranquillizers **chlorpromazine** is a well-tried drug and can be administered orally, rectally or intramuscularly but hypotension of worrying degree is not uncommon. Therefore **haloperidol** and **droperidol** are to be preferred and these also cause less drowsiness. However extrapyramidal side effects are more common and dystonic spasms are distressing both to patients and observers. When they occur they can be rapidly controlled by intramuscular or intravenous procyclidine 5–10 mg and then continued orally in a prophylactic manner.

Haloperidol can be given orally, intramuscularly or intravenously, 5–10 mg orally is given in milder cases of violence, 10–30 mg intravenously for more serious cases. Droperidol is similar but given in somewhat lower dosage.

The Burned Child

The psychological problems of the burned child are sometimes overlooked. The work of Bernstein and his colleagues at the children's burns unit has focused attention on the problems. There is a wide variety of burned children and as survival techniques improve for some there will be an increasing amount of painful suffering ahead, albeit balanced by a lessening of distress and morbidity in the less severely afflicted. A few general points are discussed.

The life events surrounding the burn may be horrific such as loss of siblings and parents and deliberate cruelty, arson, as well as ignorance or incompetence. How much opportunity is given to the child to ventilate fears and anxieties about the incident? How much is deliberately suppressed? How important is this?

Behaviour in the Unit

Regressive behaviour occurs in adults as well as children but the clinical signs in children may be less familiar for the staff concerned. Regression in a toddler will differ from the pre-pubertal child. Intermediate stages with manipulative behaviour testing the strengths and weakness of the staff, as happens with parents, are to be expected. Nearer to discharge the older child will have some foreboding of the difficulties ahead concerning deformity and malfunction and may show anxiety and depression. Staff must be alert to these phases and give support in the regressed stage. There must be understanding and perseverance with encouragement when the depressed child fails to co-operate in the rehabilitative process.

Long-term Adaptation and Outcome

In a child's favour is physical fitness, rapid healing, resilience and growth. Most children recover quite well without major psychological difficulty. Nevertheless on closer examination it is found that a proportion of children who have had major burns suffer considerably. Parents report behaviour disorders such as fears, anxiety, depression and aggression, and psychosomatic disturbances such as enuresis, sleep disturbance and feeding difficulties.

Adolescents are normally very sensitive about their changing body image. Scarring and facial disfigurement add considerably to their problems. Society at large rejects and averts from the deformed and their younger peers will be particularly disinhibited from comment. Social withdrawal and avoidance is common. Females show lowered self esteem compared with males. A few quite severely deformed appear to be able to rise above these handicaps and complete their maturational development seemingly little scathed.

Prolonged hospitalization, clinic attendances and recurrent surgery all disrupt schooling and education. This, though significant in itself, also has other effects of isolation from peers, restriction of physical and social activity, increased dependency on parents, overprotective attitudes of the parents and perhaps financial stresses for the family. In specialized burns centres which cater for children these problems are more easily identified and tackled. Where facilities for children are more occasional or scattered the problems for the child remain and their solution is more taxing.

Treatment Methods

Frequent access and visiting by parents during hospitalization and involvement of the family in the treatment and long-term rehabilitation aims are very important. The roles of the paediatrician, social service worker and child psychiatrist will vary in different units, but all have been shown to be helpful. School teachers based in hospital or from the child's school can be sought and most local education departments try to be helpful. The paediatrician may be able to advise on infant stimulation and play activities for the younger child.

Child Abuse and Non-accidental Injury

Physical abuse of children ranges from carelessness and neglect through to deliberately inflicted injury. Surgeons should look carefully at scalds and cigarette burns in children; a detailed history should be taken noting particularly inconsistency in the story, lack of concern, any discrepancy between the injury and its explanation, and delay in reporting. Other injuries, bruises, fractures, scars past and present, may be observed. The welfare of the child is paramount and admission to a place of safety, often a paediatric unit, is important. As the first observer the surgeon has an important identifying role. Paediatricians, child psychiatrists and social service departments are well versed in the statutory procedures for such cases and should be called in for advice at an early stage. Clear cases are taken to court but in some there can only be suspicion. Careful clinical notes, drawings and photography are important; careful follow-up procedures must be instituted. If the child's discharge is demanded, a magistrate's order to keep the child in hospital may be sought.

The Mentally Handicapped

The mentally handicapped are at risk. Perhaps the more dependent who are looked after by others are at less risk than those of borderline intelligence who have more chance of self care and independent existence. Most districts have a psychiatrist responsible for the welfare of this group and will know of supportive agencies.

Social Work

There are two main contributions of social work in burns care. First is technical knowledge and liaison between various social and welfare agencies. There may be urgent problems of child welfare, homelessness and bereavement at an early stage, followed by negotiation of community rehabilitative support during the recovery stage and the securing of appropriate financial benefits. The second and often more important role is the psychotherapeutic skill exercised with relatives, patients and staff. The social worker has a position outside the medical and hospital framework and this can be an advantage. Sometimes social workers have a particular skill with say children or the bereaved; such skills are often in short supply and should be readily welcomed. Hopefully, they may be encouraged to extend their interest and skills in local burns care.

Post-traumatic Neurosis and Compensation Claims

As in other trauma a proportion of the burned subsequently develop a neurotic illness. These are often characterized by mild continuing depression, loss of drive, fears and anxieties perhaps understandably linked to the burns incident, insomnia and a changed zest for life. It has been clearly shown that significant major life events can precipitate both psychosis and neurosis. There are suggestions that those with pre-existing bouts of neurotic disturbance are more at risk. Sometimes those with no previous psychological morbidity state that their lives have been permanently affected by the burns incident. These disorders appear remarkably resistant to the normal treatment measures and disproportionately disabling. The burned victim is subject not only to his own inner psychopathology but the influence of family, friends, workers, unions and employers etc.

Post-traumatic neurosis exists whether or not there are compensation issues. Whether the neurosis following the burn signifies a causal relationship cannot be tested, nor can the subject's power of control over these matters. The presence of compensation rights further complicates an already fraught subject. Undoubtedly there are a few frank malingerers consciously assuming disability in front of doctors, insurance companies and lawyers but the conscious and unconscious motivation of the vast majority are far more difficult to disentangle. The law appears to encourage simple polarization of the issues and some members of the medical profession find it easy to represent one extreme or the other. Cogent arguments for justice can be marshalled for either side. Perhaps Trimble's balanced review more adequately reflects current medical opinion than the startling revelations of Miller in his studies of accident neurosis two decades before.

Relationships with the Police

In some burns incidents the possibility of criminal acts, negligence and arson arise. Other people may have been severely injured or killed. It may be important to secure vital information quickly. The surgeon will have to judge the balance of priority between medical and surgical procedures, the patient's lucidity, the prognosis and civil responsibilities. When frank psychiatric illness is involved there may be time to get an urgent specialist opinion of the patient's capacity for interview beforehand. Additionally in such circumstances it is helpful to both the patient and the police if a senior member of staff is present throughout the interview. Attempted suicide is not a criminal act but reckless behaviour endangering other people's lives associated with such an act may be. The police do not have access to case notes but courts do.

References

BERNSTEIN, N. R. & ROBSON, M. C. (eds) (1983) *Comprehensive Approaches to the Burned Person*. Medical Examination Publishing Co., New York.

BHADHURI, R.(1982) Self-inflicted Burns. *Burns,* **8**, 403.

BOWDEN, M. L., JONES, C. A. & FELLER, I.(1984) *Psychosocial Aspects of a Severe Burn*. National Institute for Burn Medicine, Michigan.

FOWLER, J.(1978) Child Maltreatment by Burning. *Burns,* **5**, 83.

GILJOHANN, A.(1980) Adolescents Burned as Children. *Burns,* **7**, 95.

GONZALES, E. L.(1984) Psychosocial Adjustment of Children after Acute Burns. *J. Burn Care Rehab.,* **5**, 138.

IMBUS, S. & ZAWACKI, B. E.(1977) Autonomy for Burned Patients When Survival is Unprecedented. *N. Engl. J. Med.,* **297**, 308.

KUMAR, P.(1984) Child Abuse by Thermal Injury. *Burns,* **10**, 344.

MACARTHUR, J. D. & MOORE, F. D.(1975) Epidemiology of Burns. *J. Am. Med. Assoc.,* **231**, 259.

MARTIN, H. L.(1980) Psychological Effects of Accidental Injury in Childhood. *Burns,* **7**, 90.

MARZOUK, B. B., GIACALONE, T., THIEULARD, L. & WASSERMAN, D.(1982) Behavioural Changes in Burned Adult Patients. *Burns,* **8**, 365.

MILLER, H.(1961) Accident Neurosis. *Br. Med. J.,* **i**, 919 & 992.

NOYES, R., FRYE, S., SLYMEN, D. J. & CANTER, A.(1979) Stressful Live Events and Burn Injuries. *J. Trauma,* **19**, 141.

PERRY, S. & BLANK, K.(1984) Delirium in Burned Patients. *J. Burn Care Rehab.,* **5**, 210.

REST, S. M.(1984) Coping with Facial Burns. In Wachtel, T. L. and Frank, D. H. (eds) *Burns of the Head and Neck*. Saunders, Philadelphia.

TRIMBLE, M. R.(1981) *Post-traumatic Neurosis, from Railway Spine to the Whiplash*. Wiley, Chichester.

WHITE, A. C.(1982) Psychiatric Study of Patients with Severe Burns. *Br. Med. J.,* **284**, 465.

WILKINS, T. J. & CAMPBELL, J. L.(1980) Psychosocial Concerns in the Paediatric Burns Unit. *Burns,* **7**, 208.

Appendices

Normal average values

Age	Weight (kg)	Height (cm)	Blood vol (ml/kg)	Hb (g)	PCV (%)	Water requirements (ml/kg/day)	Calories (per kg/day)	Minimum Urine output(ml/hr)	Insensible loss (ml/kg)
Birth	3.5	50	85	18	61	130	112	10	31
6 months	7	65	80	11	32	120	109	10	29
1 year	10	75	75	12	36	110	105	10	27
2 years	13	86	75	13	37	102	101	15	27
3 years	15	97	72	13	38	95	98	15	26
4 years	17	104	72	13	38	93	97	15	26
5 years	19	110	72	13	39	90	96	15	25
6 years	21	115	72	13	39	86	93	20	24
7 years	23	123	72	13	40	82	90	20	23
8 years	25	131	72	13	40	78	85	20	22
9 years	28	135	72	13	41	76	80	20	21
10 years	32	140	72	14	42	75	75	25	20
12 years	40		72	14	42	70	70	25	20
14 years	50		72	14	42	60	65	30	20
16 years	55		70	14	42	50	60	35	20
Male			70	15	47	30–35	35–40	35	20
Adults Female			65	14	42	30–35	35–40	35	20

Expected normal values of urine, per 24 hours

	Metric units	Conversion factor	SI units
Creatine	0–50 mg	7.6	0–380 μmol (adult) 68 μmol (infant)
Creatinine	1–2 g	8.85	8.85–17.7 μmol
Creatinine clearance	80–120 ml/min		
Copper	10–50 μg	0.0157	0.2–0.8 mmol
Glomerular filtration rate	105–140 ml/min		
Glucose	0–0.2 g %	55.5	0–11 mmol/l
Nitrogen non-protein	10–20 g	0.0714	0.7–1.43 mmol
Osmolality	300–1000 mosmol/kg H_2O		
Potassium	30–100 mEq	1	30–100 mmol
Protein albumin	0–0.1 g		
pH	4.5–8.0		
Sodium	50–200 mEq	1	50–200 mmol
Specific gravity	1003–1030		
Urea	10–35 g	16.6	170–580 mmol
Urine output	0.5–1.0 ml/kg body weight/h		

Expected normal values of blood constituents

	Metric units	Conversion factor	SI units	Specimen bottle
Base excess	±2mEq/l	1	2 mmol/l	Lithium heparin 5 ml
Bicarbonate				
actual	22–32 mEq/l	1	22–32 mmol/l	Lithium heparin 5 ml
standard	21–25 mEq/1	1	21–25 mmol/l	Lithium heparin 5 ml
Calcium	8.5–10.5 mg %	0.25	2.2–2.6 mmol/l	Clotted 15 ml
total	4.5–5.0 mEq %			
ionized	4.0–5.0 mg %	0.25	1.0–1.25 mmol/l	Clotted 15 ml
Carbon dioxide				
$PvCO_2$	40–52 mm Hg	0.133	5.3–6.9 kPa	Heparinized 5 ml
$PaCO_2$	34–46 mm Hg	0.133	4.5–6.1 kPa	Heparinized 5 ml
content	48–52 µg %	1	48–52 µmol/l	Heparinized 5 ml
Copper	80–150 µg %	0.157	13–24 ηmol/l	Sequestrene 10 ml
Creatine	0.2–0.8 mg %	76	15.2–60.8 µmol/l	Lithium heparin 10 ml
Creatinine	0.5–1.4 mg %	88.4	45–120 µmol/l	Lithium heparin 5 ml
Fibrinogen	200–500 mg %	0.01	2.0–5.0 g/l	Citrated 10 ml
Glucose				
fasting	55–85 mg %	0.055	3.0–4.6 mmol/l	Fluoride 1 ml
post-meal	< 180 mg %	0.055	< 10 mmol/l	Fluoride 1 ml
Iron	80–160 µg %	0.179	14–30 µmol/l	Clotted 10 ml
Ketones	0.8–1.4 mg %	98	80–140 µmol/l	Lithium heparin 10 ml
Osmolality	280–300 mosmol/kg H_2O			Lithium heparin 15 ml
Phosphate	2.5–4.5 mg %	0.3	0.8–1.45 mmol/l	Clotted 15 ml

Expected normal values of blood constituents *continued*

	Metric units	Conversion factor	SI units	Specimen bottle
pH venous	7.32–7.42		38–48 nmol/l	Heparinized 5 ml
pH arterial	7.36–7.45		36–44 nmol/l	Heparinized 5 ml
PO₂ arterial	90–110 mmHg	0.133	11–15 kPa	Heparinized 5 ml
pCO₂ arterial	34–46	0.133	4.5–6.1 kPa	Heparinized 5 ml
Potassium	3.8–5.0 mEq/l	1	3.8–5.0 mmol/l	Lithium heparin 5 ml
Protein				
total	6.0–8.0 g %	10	60–80 g/l	Clotted 10 ml
albumin	3.5–5.0 g %	10	35–50 g/l	Clotted 10 ml
globulin	2.4–3.7 g %	10	24–37 g/l	Clotted 10 ml
fibrinogen	0.2–0.4 g %	10	20–40 g/l	In EDTA 5 ml
Sodium	135–148 mEq/l	1	135–148 mmol/l	Lithium heparin 5 ml
Transaminase				
SGOT	0–40 units/ml	0.75	4–18 IU/l	Clotted 5 ml
SGPT	0–12 units/ml	2.0	< 23 IU/l	Clotted 5 ml
Urea	15–40 mg %	0.166	2.5–6.5 mmol/l	Lithium heparin 5 ml
Urea nitrogen	8–20 mg %	0.166	1.33–3.3 mmol/l	Lithium heparin 5 ml
Zinc	80–120 μg %	0.154	12.2–18.4 μmol/l	Clotted 5 ml

Conversion Tables

$$\text{Millimoles/l} = \frac{10 \times \text{mg \%}}{\text{Molecular weight}} = \frac{\text{mEq/1}}{\text{Valency}}$$

$$= \frac{\text{mEq/l} \times \text{Molecular wt}}{10} = \frac{\text{mmol/l} \times \text{molecular wt}}{10}$$

$$\text{Milligrams \%} = \frac{\text{mEq/l} \times \text{Molecular wt}}{10 \times \text{valency}}$$

$$\text{Milliequivalents/l} = \frac{\text{mg \%} \times 10 \times \text{valency}}{\text{Molecular wt}} = \text{mmol/l} \times \text{valency}$$

Compound	Molecular/atomic weight	Valency
Carbon	12	2.4
Nitrogen	14	3.5
Oxygen	16	2
Sodium	23	1
Chlorine	35.5	1
Potassium	39	1
Calcium	40	1
Acetate	60	1
Bicarbonate	61	1
Lactate	90	1
Gluconate	195	1
Citrate	210	1

Conversion Tables *continued*

Length:
1 cm	= 0.394 inches	1 inch	= 2.54 cm
1 m	= 3.271 feet	1 foot	= 30.48 cm

Weight:
1 g	= 0.035 oz	1 ounce	= 28.35 g
1 kg	= 2.2 lb	1 lb	= 0.454 kg
1 kg	= 0.16 stones	1 stone	= 6.35 kg

Area:
1 cm^2	= 0.15 in^2	1 in^2	= 6.45 cm^2
1 m^2	= 10.76 ft^2	1 ft^2	= 0.093 m^2

Volume:
1 ml	= 0.035 fluid oz	1 fluid oz	= 28.42 ml
1 litre	= 1.76 pints	1 pint	= 0.568 litres = 20 fluid oz
1 litre	= 0.22 gallons	1 gallon	= 4.55 litres
1 teaspoon	= 4.5 ml	1 tablespoon	= 15 ml
1 teacup	= 120 ml	1 dessertspoon	= 8 ml
1 wineglass	= 60 ml	1 tumbler glass	= 240 ml
1 in^3	= 16387 mm^3	1 foot^3	= 0.03 m^3

Density:
1 lb/in^3	= 2.8 × 10^4 kg/m^3	1 lb/ft^3	= 16 kg/m^3

Conversion Tables *continued*

Pressure:

mmHg	cmH$_2$O	N/m^2	psi	kPa
1.0	= 1.36	= 133.3	= 0.0194	= 0.133
0.74	= 1.0	= 98.06	= 0.0143	= 0.09806
51.7	= 70.3	= 6894.76	= 1.0	= 6.895
7.50	= 10.19	= 1.0 × 10^3	= 0.146	= 1.0

Energy:

1 Joule	= 1 Newtonmetre	= 0.239 Calories
1 Calorie		= 4.19 Joules

Temperature:
To convert °C into °F, multiply by 9/5 and add 32.
To convert °F into °C, subtract 32 and multiply by 5/9

°C	°F		°C	°F
100	212		35	95
41	105.8		34	93.2
40	104		33	91.4
39	102.2		32	89.6
38	100.4		31	87.8
37	98.6		30	86
36	96.8		0	32

Equipment

The following equipment is prepared for use in the resuscitation room.

For maintaining the airway	Oral airway Anaesthetic mask BLB bag Oral suction catheters High pressure electric suction machine Oxygen administration apparatus Tongue forceps Laryngoscope Endotracheal tube Endotrachael suction catheters Bronchoscopy set Bronchoscopy suction catheters Tracheostomy set Anaesthetic machine and/or mechanical ventilator
For ensuring adequate and carefully monitored intravenous fluid replacement to correct hypovolaemic shock	Drip stand Intravenous cannulae Intravenous fluid administration set Intravenous infusion pump or burette Adhesive tape, splints and bandages for fixation of intravenous infusion equipment Intravenous cut-down set and suture material
Analgesia to prevent neurogenic shock	Morphia for intravenous use Syringe and needle suitable for intravenous drug administration Nitrous oxide ('gas and air') cylinder and administration set

To prevent the burned areas sticking to the trolley linen, so causing pain and further damage to the skin cells

A sheet of foam rubber (6 ft long × 27 in wide × ½ in thick (183 × 69 × 1.25 cm)) sprayed with silicone is placed over the casualty stretcher trolley

For careful removal and safe storage of patient's clothing, which may be required for forensic tests

Large scissors
Large plastic bag suitable to store patients clothing

For accurate measurement of urine output and early diagnosis of urine infection or other disease such as diabetes

Bladder catheterization set
Urine drainage bag suitable for very accurate assessment of hourly output and for frequent collection of samples for testing
Urine specimen bottles and forms for culture and sensitivity
Equipment for routine urine testing and specific gravity

For observation of temperature, pulse and blood pressure

Thermometer
Watch or clock with second hand
Stethoscope
Sphygmomanometer

For diagnosis and assessment of patient's requirements during the burn resuscitation period

Syringes and needles suitable for venepuncture
Laboratory forms and specimen bottles for:
haemoglobin
haematocrit (packed cell volume)
serum electrolytes
blood urea
cross-matching
carboxyhaemoglobin
blood gases (have heparin available)

For emergency surgery to relieve constricture of neck, chest and limbs in deep circumferential burns	Sterile surgical gloves Scalpel and No.10 blades Large gauze swabs (abdominal size) Sterile saline for topical use (minimum 1 litre)
For dressing wounds to prevent further damage to the skin and infection	Sterile gloves Limb size sheets of foam rubber (¼in (0.6 cm) thick) sprayed with silicone Sterile Kling film Sterile vaseline gauze Sterile gauze swabs (abdominal size) Sterile cotton wool Bandages Adhesive tape Sharp-pointed scissors Bandage scissors Dressing forceps
To diagnose and prevent damage to cornea if the eyelids are burnt	Hypromellose artificial tears or saline eye drops Fluorescein eye drops Sterile saline for eye irrigation Undine Chloramphenicol eye ointment
To take swabs from nose, throat, rectum and the burn sites for early detection of infection	Wound swabs and transport media Laboratory forms for microbiology

Admission pack

2 Curved heavy Aufrichts scissors
2 Straight heavy Aufrichts scissors
4 McIndoe non-toothed dressing
    forceps
4 Heavy plain dressing forceps

2 Iris scissors
2 Bandage scissors 7 in (17 cm)
2 Mayo scissors 7 in (17 cm)
5 Curved Dunhill artery forceps on
    pin

To set up theatre

Damp dust all services
3 Trolleys needed

Burns set★
5 Large towel packs
1 Bowl set plus 1–2 extra bowls
Diathermy forceps and quiver
    (check pad is on patient)
5 Skin graft blades
3 Scalpel blades
3 Sutures – surgeon's choice
6 in (15 cm) Crepe bandages – for
    trunks and above knee
4 in (10 cm) Crepe bandages – for
    arms and below knee
7–8 paper dressing sheets
Extra lap sheets
1 Pack 18 × 18 Raytecs (25) (May
    need a pack of 50 for large ops)
    (Adult)

1 Pack 12 × 12 Raytecs (25) (May
    need a pack of 50 for large ops)
    (Child)
3 Packs of 4 × 3 Raytecs
Leg dressings (3 for one whole leg)★
2 Packs of surgeon's gowns
2 Packs of nail brushes
4 Liquid paraffin
12 Chlorhexidine gluconate★ – for
    cleaning
Paranet – Cut into 8in (20 cm) strips
    or spread onto leg dressings
Additional instruments according to
    surgeon's preference or specific
    requests.

★If a large operation a Burns Extra
    Pack may be needed

To have ready if needed

Skin mesher with Dermacarriers
Esmarch bandages for limbs

Skin jar
Hot saline in hot cabinet

Burn sets

5 Lanes tissue forceps
10 Large curved artery forceps
10 Mosquito forceps
10 Bachaus towel clips
2 Bandage scissors
2 Mayo scissors
2 Aufricht's scissors (straight heavy)
2 Aufricht's scissors (curved heavy)
2 Strabismus scissors (COF)
2 Iris scissors

2 No.3 BP handles
1 No.4 BP handle
1 Barron's knife handle
2 Adson's toothed dissecting forceps
2 Adson's non-toothed dissecting
    forceps
2 Gillies' toothed dissecting forceps
6 McIndoe's dissecting forceps
2 Heavy plain dressing forceps
2 Lane's toothed dissecting forceps

Burn sets *Continued*

1 McIndoe's scissors
1 Howarth elevator
1 Ruler
1 Chip syringe
3 Sinus forceps
3 Rampley sponge holders
1 Large skin board
2 Small skin boards

2 Allis tissue forceps
1 Volkmanns spoon
1 Pen with nib
1 Ink pot
3 Nevert needle holders
1 Russell Davies desloughing forceps
4 Watson knives

Burns extra set

1 Watson desloughing knife
1 Watson graft knife
4 Rampley sponge holding forceps
1 6 in (15 cm) ruler

1 Bandage scissors
1 Iris scissors
1 Strabismus scissors

Plastic set

1 Barron's handle
2 No. 3 BP Handles
1 No. 4 BP Handle
2 McIndoe forceps (non-toothed)
1 Gillies' forceps (toothed)
1 Adson's forceps (toothed)
1 Lane's forceps (toothed and heavy)
1 McIndoe's scissors
1 Aufricht's scissors (curved and heavy)
1 Aufricht's scissors (straight and heavy)
1 Aufricht's scissors (curved and fine)
1 Aufricht's scissors (straight and fine)
1 Iris scissors
1 Strabismus scissors
1 Small curved scissors
2 Gillies' skin hooks (long)
2 Kilner skin hooks
2 Joseph's double skin hooks
2 Cats paw retractors

1 Desmarres retractor (small)
1 Kilner retractor (small)
1 American pattern sucker
1 7 in (18 cm) Mayo scissors
1 Cartridge syringe
10 Bachaus towel clips (5 small, 5 large)
10 Mosquito artery forceps (5 curved, 5 straight on pin)
1 Plastic tray
1 Sponge
1 Small gallipot
1 Large gallipot
1 Nevert's needle holder
3 Rampley's sponge holders
1 Tilley's nasal forceps
1 Sinus forceps
1 Derf needle holder
1 Howarth elevator
1 6 in (15 cm) ruler
1 Mapping pen with nib
1 Ink pot

Skin mesher

Mesher
Handle

Sterilization case
Allen key

Davies dermatome

1 Miniplex Davies Dermatome
1 Simplex Davies Dermatome

1 Duplex Davies Dermatome
1 Drive shaft

Theatre bowl sets

1 14 in (35 cm) Bowl
2 6½ in (16 cm) Metal bowls
2 4½ in (12 cm) Metal bowls
1 3½ in (9 cm) Plastic gallipot

2 3 in (7 cm) Metal gallipots
1 10 in (25 cm) Plastic receiver
2 8 in (20 cm) Metal receivers
1 6 in (15 cm) Metal receiver

Dressing instrument sets

1 Curved heavy Aufricht's scissors
1 Straight Aufrichts scissors
2 McIndoe's non-toothed dressing
   forceps

2 Heavy plain dressing forceps
1 Iris scissors

Paracentesis set

1 Trocar and cannula, 16 fg
1 Trocar and cannula, 21 fg
1 Gate clip

1 No. 4 Bard Parker handle
1 18 in (45 cm) PC rubber tubing
   5 mm

Ophthalmic pack

Set of lacrymal probes
1 Iris scissors
1 McIndoe dressing forceps

2 Desmarre retractors
1 Iris forceps
1 Glass undine

Steinmann pin set

1 Large stirrup
1 Small stirrup
2 Traction loops
2 Bowler caps
2 Spacers
2 Ends
2 Small Spencer wells
Steinmann pins 6 in (15 cm) × 4 mm

Steinmann pins 9 in
   (22.5 cm) × 4 mm
3 Rampley sponge holding forceps
1 No. 3 scalpel handle
1 Barsky dissecting forceps
1 Plain heavy dressing forceps
1 Lanes dissecting forceps
1 Universal handle with Jacob chuck
1 Large pair wire cutters

Theatre catheter tray

1 Large receiver
2 Small gallipots
1 Penile clamp

1 Disposable gallipot
2 Spongeholders
10 Green swabs

Tracheostomy set

1 No. 3 Bard Parker handle
1 No. 4 Bard Parker handle
1 Mastoid retractor wests 5½ in
  (14 cm)
2 Allis tissue forceps
2 Spongeholders
2 Mosquito forceps, curved
6 Mosquito forceps, straight
6 Dunhill artery forceps
2 Double blunt hooks
1 Tilley's nasal forceps
3 Towel clips
1 Toothed dissecting forcep, Treves
1 TOE dissecting forcep
1 Waugh's dissecting forcep,
  toothed

1 Waugh's dissecting forcep, plain
2 Needle holders
1 Mayo scissor, straight 6½ in
  (16 cm)
1 McIndoe's scissors
1 Stitch scissors
1 Self-clearing suction tube
1 Yankauer's suction tube
1 Tracheal dilator
3 Jacques catheters (1 × 8 fg,
  1 × 10 fg, 1 × 12 fg)
3 Gallipots, polypropylene
3 Silver tracheostomy tubes
  (1 × 18 fg, 1 × 24 fg, 1 × 26 fg)
1 4 in (10 cm) Bowl, polypropylene
1 Receiver, polypropylene

Bone set

1 Farabeuf's Rugine (flat)
1 Farabeuf's Rugine (curved)
1 Horsley bone cutter
1 Liston bone cutter
1 McIndoe bone cutter
2 Bone nibblers
3 Osteotomes
3 Gouges
1 Heath mallet

1 Amputation saw
1 Amputation guard
1 Rasp
1 Sequestrum forcep
1 Bone forcep
5 Large Spencer Wells artery forceps
1 Volkmann spoon
1 McIndoe bone hook
1 Langenbeck 21.5 cm retractor

Hospitals with Burn Facilities in Great Britain and Ireland

The details given below were correct at the time of going to press.

Regional Health Authority	Hospitals	Telephone No.
Northern	Newcastle General, Westgate Road, Newcastle-on-Tyne NE4 6BE	Newcastle (0632) 738811
	Sick Children's Great North Road, Newcastle NE2 3A2	Newcastle (0632) 816177
	Middlesbrough General, Ayresome Green Lane, Middlesbrough, Cleveland TS5 5AZ	Middlesbrough (0642) 813133
	Shotley Bridge General Shotley Bridge, Consett, Co. Durham	Consett (0207) 503456
North Western	Booth Hall Chidren's, Charleston Road, Blackley, Manchester M9 2AA	Manchester (061) 7957000
	Withington, Nell Lane, West Didsbury, Manchester M20 8LE	Manchester (061) 445 8111
Mersey	Whiston, Prescot, Merseyside L35 5DR	Liverpool (051) 426 1600
	Alder Hey Childrens, Eaton Road, Liverpool L12 2AP	Liverpool (051) 228 4811
Yorkshire	Pinderfields, Wakefield, West Yorks.	Wakefield (0924) 375217

Regional Health Authority	*Hospitals*	*Telephone No.*
Trent	Leicester Royal Infirmary, Leicester LE1 5WW	Leicester (0533) 541414
	Nottingham City, Hucknall Road, Nottingham NG5 1PB.	Nottingham (0602) 608111
	Fulwood, Sheffield S10 3TD	Sheffield (0742) 302971
West Midlands	Birmingham Accident, Bath Row, Birmingham B15 1NA	Birmingham (021) 643 7041
Oxford	Stoke Mandeville, Aylesbury, Bucks 4P21 8AL	Aylesbury (0296) 84111
East Anglian	West Norwich, Bowthorpe Road, Norwich, Norfolk	Norwich (0606) 28377
North West Thames	Mount Vernon, Northwood, Middlesex	Northwood (09274) 26111
North East Thames	St Andrews, Billericay, Essex	Billericay (02774) 22611
	University College Hospital, Gower Street, London, WC1E 6AU	London (01) 387 9300
South East Thames	Queen Victoria, East Grinstead, Sussex	East Grinstead (0342) 24111
	Queen Elizabeth Military, London SE18	London (01) 856 5533
	Guy's Hospital, London SE1 9RT	London (01) 407 7600
South West Thames	Queen Mary's, Roehampton, London SW15	London (01) 789 6611

Regional Health Authority	Hospitals	Telephone No.
Wessex	Odstock, Salisbury, Wiltshire SP2 8BJ	Salisbury (0722) 6262
South Western	Frenchay, Bristol BS16 1LE	Bristol (0272) 565656
	Derriford, Plymouth, Devon	Plymouth (0752) 777111
Wales	St Lawrence, Chepstow, Gwent	Chepstow (02912) 2334
Scotland: Grampian	Royal Infirmary Aberdeen AB9 2ZB	Aberdeen (0224) 681818
Glasgow	Royal Infirmary, Glasgow G4 0SF	Glasgow (041) 552 3535
Lothian	Bangour General, Broxburn, W.Lothian EH52 6LR	Dechmont (050681) 334
Edinburgh	Royal Hospital for Sick Children Edinburgh EH9 1LF	Edinburgh (031) 667 1991
Tayside	Dundee Royal Infirmary, Barrack Road, Dundee	Dundee (0382) 23125
Ireland	Royal Victoria, Grosvenor Road, Belfast BT12 6BA	Belfast (0232) 240503
	Cork Regional, Wilton, Cork	Cork (21) 46400
	Dr Steevens Steevens Lane Dublin 8	Dublin (0001) 772606

Poison Centres for Advice

(Only for use by Medical Practitioners)

The details given below were corrrect at the time of going to press.

London	New Cross Hospital, London SE14 5BH	Tel: 01 635 9191
Cardiff	Ambulance HQ St Fagan's Road, Cardiff	Tel: 0222 569200
Edinburgh	Royal Infirmary, Edinburgh EH3 9YW	Tel: 031 229 2477
Birmingham	Dudley Road Hospital, Birmingham B18 7QH	Tel: 021 554 3801 Ext. 4123
Belfast	Royal Victoria Hospital Belfast BT12 6BA	Tel: 0232 240503 Ext. 2140
Dublin	Jervis Street Hospital, Dublin	Tel: 0001 723355
Newcastle	Royal Victoria Hospital, Queen Victoria Road, Newcastle NE1 4LP	Tel: 0632 325131
Manchester	Booth Hall Hospital, Charlestown Road, Blackley, Manchester M9 2AA	Tel: 061 795 7000

European Association of Poison Control Centres, P.O. Box 1057, Blindern, Oslo, Norway. Tel: 2/46 51 27.

US National Clearing House for Poison Control Centres, Bureau of Drugs, Room 1346, 5600 Fishers Lane, Rockville, Maryland 20857, USA.

International Poison Advice Centres

Country	Address and Telephone Number	
Australia	Royal Canberra Hospital, Acton, ACT 2601.	Tel: 62 43 2111
Austria	I Med Univ Klinik, Spitelgasse 23, 1090 Wien.	Tel: 222/434343
Belgium	Rue Joseph Stallaert 1 B15, 1060 Brussels.	Tel: (0) 2/3 454545
Canada	Hospital for Sick Children, 555 University Avenue, Toronto M5G 1X8.	Tel: 416/597 1500 ext. 1505

Country	Address and Telephone Number	
Czechoslovakia	Vysehradsky 49, Praha 2.	Tel: 2/293868
Denmark	Opgang 7301, Tagensvej 20, 2200 Copenhagen N.	Tel: (0) 1/394233
Finland	University Hospital, Stenbäckinkatu 11, 00290 Helsinki 29.	Tel: 0/4711 2788
France	Hôpital Fernand Widal, 200 Rue du Faubourg St Denis, 75475 Paris.	Tel: 1/4205 6329
Germany	Spandauer Damm 130, 1000 Berlin 19.	Tel: (0) 30/30 35466
Greece	Childrens Hospital, 'Aglaia Kyriakou', 11527 Athens.	Tel: (0) 1 7793777
Hungary	Hôpital Sandor Koranya, Alsoerdosor 7, 1074 Budapest.	Tel: 1/223450
Italy	Policlinico Umberto I, Via del Policlinico, 00161 Roma.	Tel: (0) 6/490663
Netherlands	Antonie van Leeuwenhoikl 9, Postbus 3720 BA, Bilthoven.	Tel: (0) 30/742200
Norway	Farmakologisk Institutt, Odontolobygningen, PO Box 1057, Blindern, 0316 Oslo 3.	Tel: 2/465127
New Zealand	Otago Medical School, PO Box 913, Dunedin.	Tel: 740 999 ext. 8345
Poland	Szpital Praski III, Al Swierczewskiego 67, 03-701 Warszawa.	Tel: 1/190897
Portugal	Rue Infante D Pedro 8, 1700 Lisboa.	Tel: 19/761176
Rumania	Calea Floreasca 8, Bucresti.	Tel: 79 40 65
Spain	Farmacia 9, Madrid 4.	Tel: 1/232 3366
Sweden	Karolinska Sjukhuset, PO Box 60500, 10401 Stockholm.	Tel: (0) 8/33 1231
Switzerland	Klosbachstrasse 107, 8030 Zurich.	Tel: (0) 1/2515151
Turkey	Cemel Gürsel Cad No 18, Sihhiye-Ankara.	Tel: (41) 337000
Yugoslavia	University Centre, Zaloska 7, 61000 Ljubljana.	Tel: (61) 31 42 66 ext. 23–55

Index

Accident/emergency department
    management 24–40
    airway 24–5
    analgesia 25
    assessment of burn 29–31
    bleeding 25
    examination 26–7
    eyelids 38
    history 26
    preparation for arrival 24
    records 26–7
    shock 25–6
    transfer from 28–9
    wound cleaning 33
Acetic acid 74
Acid-base equilibrium 57–8
Admission procedures 39
Adult respiratory distress
    syndrome 138
Aeroplane splint 194–6
Aetiology 4–5
Air-fluidized bed 72
Albumin, serum 138
Alcoholism 223
    delirium due to 224
Alkali burns 20, 93
Ammonium hydroxide burns 93
Anaesthesia 115–24
    airway 116
    children 119–21
    dressings/minor procedures 122
    drugs 116–17
    excision/grafting
        procedures 115–19
    late complications of burns 124
    monitoring during 119
    premedication 115–16
Analgesia 25, 75, 117
Ankle
    scar/contracture, prevention/
        minimizing 169
    splint 207, 208 (figs.)
Anoxia 128 (table)
Antecubital fossa contracture 183
Axilla
    contracture 183, 184 (fig.)
    splint 194–6

Bactigras 69
Barbiturate dependence 224
Bath therapy 74
Bitumen burns 20, 96, 97 (fig.)
Blood constituents, expected
    normal values 240–1
Blood transfusion 48, 118
    children 120–1
    massive, complications of 118–
        19
Body weight 165 (table)
Bronchial burns 98
Burns team 211–14
    joint discussion 229
    nursing team 212–14
    stress in 229
Burns theatre 216
Burns unit 214–17
    heating 214
    infection control 214–15
    interior design 215
    location 216–17
    space 215

Calcium oxide (lime) burns 93
Capillary nail test 28 (fig.)
Carbolic acid (phenol) burns 95–6
Carbon monoxide poisoning 126
Central venous pressure 66
Chemical burns 6, 91–9
    first aid 19–20
    ingested chemicals 20
Children *see* Paediatric patients
Chlorhexidine 72–3
Chromic acid burns 93
Circulation changes 13–14
Clinical depth of burn 13
Clinical psychologist 220
Clotting abnormalities 118–19
Compensation claims 234
Compression garments 171, 190
Consent to treatment in mentally
    ill 221
Contractures 167–74
    prevention/minimizing 167–9
    treatment 173
    see also individual structures

Conversion tables   242–4
Cooking fat burns   96
Cresol (lysol) burns   95–6
Cyanide   20

Death, approaching   225–6
Deformity/disfigurement, coping
    with   225
Delirium   223–4
    alcoholic   224
Depression   224–5
Disseminated intravascular
    coagulation   80–1
District General Hospital, early care
    in   43–51
    blood transfusion   48
    intravenous fluids   45–6, 47
    (figs.), 49 (table)
    reassessment of burn injury   43–
    4, 48, 50
    urine examination   44–5, 50
    wound cleaning   44
    wound dressing/exposure   44
Domestic precautions   9
Dressing   44
Dressing room   74–5
Drug dependence problems   222–
    3, 224

Ears   176
Elbow
    scars/contractures, prevention/
        minimizing   168
    splint   196–7
Electrical burns   6–7, 83–9, 123
    care of   88
    electric arc   87–8
    first aid   21
    high tension injuries   86–7, 88
    lightning burns   88
    low tension injuries   85–6, 88
Enteral nutrition   163 (table)
Equipment   245–51
    admission pack   248
    bone set   251
    burn extra set   249
    burn sets   248–9
    Davies dermatome   249
    dressing instrument sets   250
    ophthalmic pack   250

paracentesis set   250
plastic set   249
skin mesher   249
Steinmann pin set   250
theatre bowl sets   250
theatre catheter tray   250
to have ready if needed   248
to set up theatre   248
tracheostomy set   251
Escharectomy   106–10
Escharatomy   36–7, 122
Eye, chemical burn   20, 94
Eyebrows, late surgery   181–2
Eyelids   38, 176, 180

Face   177
Family of burned patient   227–8
Fentanyl   117, 121
First aid   18–23
    chemical burn   18–20
        eye   20
    electrical burn   21
    flame burn   18–19
    hot fluids/scalds   18
    inhalation injury   21–2
Flame burn   6, 18–19
Flash burn   6
Fluid loss   13–14, 52
Fluid replacement   117–18
Foam mattress   72
Foot, dorsum of   184
Formic acid burn   93
Frostbite   22

Gastro-intestinal tract   16
Glucose/insulin regime   80
Grafts   76–8
    application   110
    cutting split skin   108 (fig.)
    full/partial thickness   110–11
    mesh   111, 112 (fig.), 113 (figs.)
    operation   108–10
    postage-stamp   109 (fig.), 112–
        14
    pre-operative preparation
        107–8
    scar/contracture, prevention/
        minimizing   167–9
        ambulation   169
        joint movement   169

sheet 111
storage 110
timing 105–6

Haemodialysis 146–8
complications 148
vascular access 147–8
Haemoglobinuria 45 (fig.), 144–5
Hand 175
late surgery 184–5
palmar burn 186
scar/contracture, minimizing/
prevention 167–8
splint 200–7
banjo 185 (fig.), 186
dorsum 200–2, 203 (fig.)
oyster 205–7
volar surface 201 (figs.), 202–
7
Heart 15
Heat loss 14
History of burns treatment 1–3
Hospitals with burns facilities, Great
Britain & Ireland 252–4
Hydrochloric acid burns 91–2
Hydrofluoric acid burns 20, 92–3
Hyperkalaemia 56, 145
Hyperthermia 81
Hypocalcaemia 56
Hypokalaemia 56–7
Hypovolaemia 25–6

Incidence 4–5, 6 (fig.), 7 (fig.)
Infection 67–8
Inhalation burn 7
blood gas investigation 139–40
central venous pressure
measurement 140–1
chest X-ray 139
complications
adult respiratory distress
syndrome 138
low serum albumin 138
respiratory infection 136–8
fibreoptic bronchoscopy 140
first aid 21–2
hypoxaemia 125–7
intensive care 125–42
management 129–36, 137 (table)
drugs 133–4, 136

endotracheal intubation
130–2
humidification 130
intermittent positive pressure
ventilation 132–5
oxygen therapy 129–30
physiotherapy 130
positive end expiratory
pressure 135
Swan-Ganz catheterization
141
tracheostomy 132
thermal/chemical injury 125–6
Inpatient management 33
Intermittent positive pressure
ventilation 132–5
Intravenous fluids 34–6, 45–6, 47
(fig.), 49 (table), 56 (table)

Keloids 172–3
Ketamine 122, 124
Kidney 15
Knee splint 198

Laboratory investigations 34
Lightning injuries 88–9
Limbs, scars/contractures,
prevention/minimizing 167
Lime (calcium oxide) burns 93
Lithium
metallic, burns due to 20, 95
salts 223
Little finger extension splint 202,
204 (fig.), 205 (fig.)
Lungs 16–17; *see also* inhalation
burn
Lysol (cresol) burn 95–6

Management
doctor's surgery 41–2
inpatient 33
outpatient 41–2
see also District General Hospital
Mafenide acetate
(Sulphamylon) 73
Mediscus Low Air Loss Bed 72
Mental Health Act 221
Mental Health Officer 220
Mental Health team 219–20
Mentally handicapped patients 233

Mortality   8, 9 (fig.)
Mouth   176–7, 182
Muscle relaxants   117
Myoglobinuria   145

Neck   177, 178 (fig.)
    collar   191–4
    scar/contracture, prevention/
        minimizing   169, 183
    splint   191–2
Nitric acid burn   91–2
Non-survivable burns   225–6
Normal average values   238
Nose, late surgery   182–3
Nuclear explosion   102–4
Nursing team   212–14
Nutrition   158–66
    energy requirements   159 (table)
    enteral   164 (table)
    food
        composition   160–2 (table)
        weights and measures   160
            (table)
    milk   163 (table)
    minimum requirements,
        average   162 (table)
    nitrogen requirements   159
        (table)

Occlusive dressings   68–9
Oesophageal burn   96–9
Operating theatre   105–14
Oxygen therapy   129–30

Paediatric dosage   156
Paediatric patients   150–7
    abused   233
    anaesthesia   119–21
    blood transfusion   120–1
    co-operation   151–2
    cosmetic needs   154–5
    emotional needs   153
    needs of parents/family   155
    non-accidental injury   155–6,
        233
    nutritional needs   154
    physical responses/needs   151
    psychological problems   231–3
    psychological trauma   152–3
Pain relief   123

Pancuronium   117, 121
Percentages, relative, of different
    parts of body   30 (fig.), 32
    (fig.)
Peritoneal dialysis   148–9
Petrol burn   95–6
Phenoxyethanol   74
Phenol (carbolic acid) burn   95–6
Phosphorus burn   20, 95
Picric acid burn   93
Poison centres   255–6
Police, relationship with   235
Popliteal fossa
    contracture   183
    scar/contracture, prevention/
        minimizing   169
Positive end expiratory
    pressure   135
Post-operative care   119
Post-traumatic neurosis   234
Potassium, metallic, burn   93
Potassium hydroxide burn   93
Potassium permanganate burn   96
Potassium replacement   57
Prevention of burns   8–9
Proflavine wool preparation   180–1
Protein balance   16
Psychiatric aspects   218–35
Psychiatric illness   218, 221, 222–5
Psychiatrist   220
Psychological support   226–7
Psychotropic drug
    continuation   222

Radiation burn   100–4
Radiation syndrome, acute   100–2
Red cells   15
Renal failure, acute   143–9
    management   145–6
        haemodialysis *see*
            Haemodialysis
        peritoneal dialysis   148–9
    prevention   144
Replacement fluids,
    alternative   58–62
    Birmingham formula   61
    dextran 6% in saline   58
    Odstock formula   61
    Ringer's lactate   58–60
    Roehampton formula   60–1

Respiratory burns *see* Inhalation
  burns

Scalds 6, 18
Scars 167–74
  hypertrophic 170–2
  long-standing 173
  malignant change 173
  prevention/minimizing 167–9
Septicaemia 78–81
Shock 25–6
  nurse monitoring/charting 63–6
Shoulder, scar/contracture,
  prevention/minimizing 169
Sick cell syndrome 79
Silver nitrate solution 73–4
Silver sulphadiazine 73
Skin 11–12
  grafts *see* Grafts
  pathophysiological changes 12–
    13
Smoke inhalation 126
Social work 233–4
Sodium, metallic, burn 20, 95
Sodium depletion 55
Sodium hydroxide burn 93
Sodium hypochlorite burn 94
Splinting 188–210
  aeroplane 194–6
  aftercare 190–1
  ankle 207, 208 (figs.)
  axilla 194–6
  banjo 185 (fig.), 186
  dynamic 188
  elbow 196–7
  equipment 190
  exercise with 190
  hand *see under* Hand
  indications 188
  knee 198
  materials 189
  neck 191–4

oyster 205–7
preparation for theatre 107
static 189
suppliers 209
wrist 198–200
Sulphamylon (mafenide
  acetate) 73
Sulphuric acid burn 20, 93
Surface area estimation 53, 54
  (fig.)
Suxamethonium 116–17, 121

Tannic acid burn 93
Tie-over dressing 180, 181 (fig.)
Toes 184
Toxic shock 79
Transportation 22–3
Trilene burn 95–6
Tubocurarine 117

Urine, expected normal values, per
  24 hours 239

Violent patient 230–1

Water and electrolyte
  depletion 54–7
Wound care (management) 41–2,
  68–78
  circumferential burn 72
  deep burn 76
  ear 72
  exposed wound 69
  face 70
  feet 70–1
  full thickness burn 69, 76
  hand 70, 71 (fig.)
  initial cleaning 68
  occlusive dressing 68–9
  partial thickness burn 69, 75
Wound cleaning 33
Wrist splint 198–200

NOTES

NOTES

NOTES

NOTES

NOTES

NOTES

NOTES

NOTES

NOTES

NOTES